Cherubini, Diabetes Obesity

Walk Away From Diabetes and Obesity

Common Sense Diabetes Care
And
Weight Control

A Doctor's plan

How to Attach your Mind to your Body. A revolutionary approach to losing weight, controlling adult-onset diabetes, reducing its complications and living longer.

by
Thomas D. Cherubini MD

Dedication

In addition to the readers of this book, who struggle against diabetes and obesity, this book is also dedicated to my wife Fabiola, for her loyalty, her unfailing good humor, and steady encouragement.

Acknowledgements

I would like to thank my wife Fabiola, for her help in the preparation of the manuscript. Her support, patience and encouragement were indispensable. If there is anything even faintly artistic about this book, it was entirely her doing and none of my own. She also contributed several delicious, low-calorie recipes.

My son Chris, a fount of good ideas and common-sense, rendered indispensable formatting assistance, and was always there for me as well, when I needed his legal guidance, (although I didn't always take his conservative advice, much to his consternation).

I would also like to thank my friend, Peter Farrell, for suggesting the title, and friends all, the other members of the STAR investment group; Ed Andrus, Phil Bowers, Norm Keller, and Frank Nairne, for their enthusiasm and encouragement.

Preface

If you have diabetes or have been told to reduce your body weight because you might be at risk for the disease, I'm sure this is not the first book you've seen on the subject. Medical authorities agree that obesity is one of the chief causes of the rapid increase in the incidence of Type II diabetes. Over two-thirds of all Americans are overweight. In order to stave off diabetes and its attendant complications, it is universally accepted that if you are overweight or obese, losing weight is a necessity. Hence the plethora of books, TV plans, magic capsules, and exercise machines. Why are there so many?

Unfortunately, it is because most weight-loss programs do not work. If you want proof, watch television. It is almost impossible to browse the channels without coming across two or three wonderful new plans, complete with pills, machines, diet sheets, and attractive, happy people endorsing the program. And of course, the unreadable little disclaimer that the "satisfied users" do not represent the typical result. Because most of them fail in the long run, new ones are introduced continually. And they are just as ineffective. How can they get away with it? My Italian grandmother used to say, "Money makes the blind see."

So when I sat down to prepare this book, I had to ask, "Does the world need another diabetes/weight control book?" After seeing the calorie-counting emphasis of most books on the subject, and the evident lack of understanding of where the weight-control solution really lies, the answer turned out to be yes.

"Yes" because this book is different. It presumes to change not just your weight and conditioning, but *your mind.* To help you adopt and make part of yourself the mindset that is the real secret to getting thin and staying that way. Through this book, I hope to open up a better world for you, to offer you a chance to reach for the active life of good health that is our birthright. In the pages that follow is a reasoned appeal to the love of life and good health that abides in all of us. It explains how putting that love to work for us will help to illuminate the understanding we need to re-prioritize our lives. It worked for me. I am confident that it will for you, too.

Dr. T. D. Cherubini, New York City, 2010

Table of Contents

1

Introduction

The first part of this book is about a narrow escape—mine in fact. An escape from a life shortened by diabetic complications and coronary artery disease. I want to tell you about it so that you might gain from my experience and not suffer the same close call that I had. Although I am a medical doctor and should know better, I made the same mistakes we all do, because I suffer from a malady nearly all of us share. A feeling of invulnerability. A sense of "it won't, it can't happen to me." Unfortunately, under the conditions we will be discussing in this book, this denial, while useful in some other areas of our lives, in the case of attending to our health and fitness, is a psychological mechanism that soothes and protects our minds at the expense of our life span. A fascinating aspect of this erroneous belief is that it is present even when we are already sick, or physically unfit to the point of impending total breakdown of our physiological systems.

In short, it is an inability to accept the fact that each one of us is going to die. And without acknowledgment, and conscious acceptance of that universal destiny and re-adjustment of our own priorities and life-style, it will be sooner rather than later. I know I'm hitting you hard right up front, but it's not because I am cruel or uncaring. It's precisely because I do care.

Because I went through it myself, and because I am a doctor, I hope that I can help you understand the mistakes I made, and not only help you avoid them, but help you get your life back on track if you're about to stumble, or have already developed diabetes, or have a weight problem that has not responded to ordinary methods.

It isn't as though the mistakes we make are huge, thundering boulders, crashing our lives down the mountainside toward doom. They're mostly little every day lapses brought on by unquestioning acceptance of established authority, and by ignorance. And yes, by a little bit of gluttony, which, common though it is in our society, shouldn't be excusable because of it. "Everybody does it" should never be an argument.

Even if you fit this discouraging picture, you've got a leg up on me. I don't have any excuses. As a professional in health care, I'm supposed to understand these things well enough to avoid the pitfalls. But having fallen as I did only goes to prove the truth of the old observation that there's a big difference between intellectually understanding an issue and emotional acceptance of it. Like nearly all of us, I had the first, but not the second.

As I discovered to my dismay, it's not enough to "know" that you have diabetes, or a weight problem, or high cholesterol. If we are unable to accept it down deep where we live, we will never have the courage to do the things we have to do to mend our bodies and our lives. You might be astonished at how many of us are in that exact fix.

On the other hand, maybe you wouldn't be surprised at all. Obesity, high cholesterol, and adult-onset diabetes are trumpeted on every magazine cover today. They have assumed worldwide importance. And why wouldn't they have? According to recent figures, there are more than twenty-six million adult-onset diabetics in the United States, and another forty-five million pre-diabetics. The average American consumes 150 pounds of sugar annually. To do the arithmetic and put this into perspective, every American

—each man, woman and child of us, eats, in one form or another, three pounds of sugar each and every week of the year.

I have a lot to share. I hope I won't preach or moralize, and I'll try not to confuse you with arcane medical terms. I don't believe it helps understanding to be able to know whether blood glucose is measured in milligrams per deciliter, or pounds per barrelful. Sometimes, a simple number is all that is necessary, because as far as we are concerned, its usefulness is to be able to compare it to a previous value or a known standard. Most of us know that a blood sugar of 160 is above the normal upper limit of 110. Isn't that enough for understanding the concept and putting the information to use? So after the first explanation, you won't see too many units of measurement in this book.

And you will read about my enthusiasm, albeit tempered, for what some—nay, many in my profession, dismiss as "fringe" medicine—vitamins and food supplements.

"Ah yes, vitamins," doctors say thoughtfully, with hand on chin, trying to be polite.

But I understand how they feel. It makes doctors uneasy that until very recently, over-the-counter supplements have not been tested for efficacy in the reliable, traditional method of employing a double-blind study, a method in which neither the randomized volunteers, nor the scientist conducting the study, know which individual is receiving the drug, and which the placebo. (That's why it's *double-blind.*)

The double blind approach presumes to inject into the outcome the least possible influence of sponsor, tester or subject. A time-proven method to be sure, and one that if the testing sample is random enough, separates the effective from the ineffective, the safe from the dangerous. Given of course, that the testing itself spans a long enough time period, and involves a statistically adequate number of test subjects.

But despite the fact that most vitamin supplements are

roundly dismissed by many medical practitioners, many of these so-called "fringe" therapies work too, and work well. As a result, they are slowly making their way into mainstream medical practice. And legitimate research is finally beginning to show up in medical journals. In nearly every community you can find a medical doctor who has taken post-graduate courses, and specializes in nutritional and preventative medicine.

Unfortunately, the bulk of mainstream money that is provided for testing medicaments still follows the chance for profit. We live in a relatively free society after all, where business firms have to answer to their stockholders. Why would a drug company spend a lot of money to develop and test a substance from which it has no hope of ever making a dime?

In preparing this book, I re-examined a lot of material about diabetes, obesity and heart disease. I dug into the medical literature, old and new journal articles and reviews, physiology texts, and books for the general public. In these last, I noticed that it is common for writers to lard their efforts with dire statistics about the increasing incidence of diabetes in the United States, (indeed, in nearly all the countries of the civilized world as well), and with warnings about our children. They can sound like the end of the world is coming. Maybe they hope that the terrible numbers will frighten people into doing the right thing. And although I try to refrain, the numbers are so alarming that I find myself including them in my own writing.

But in fact, scare tactics never work. If you want irrefutable proof, the next time you're in the checkout line at the food market take a look around. See what the fattest Americans have in their carts. They read these books too. Among other things, it illustrates the power that advertising has over the reasoning process. We are clobbered with TV and magazine ads for sugary soda water and junk food that feature handsome men and beautiful women having the time of their lives, seemingly thanks to the sponsor's product.

The advertising must be effective. According to the American Beverage Association (ABA), in the United States alone, the soda pop business grosses more than $60 billion every year. That's $60 billion, with a "B". According to the ABA, over the 12 months of the year 2002, (The latest year for which I could obtain sales statistics. The ABA is understandably secretive about these frightening numbers.), Americans consumed 52.4 gallons of carbonated soda per person—a gallon of soda water a week. *That's almost two cans of soda every day of the year for every living soul in the United States, including children and babies.* And the amount has been increasing every year.

However true or alarming, how can dry statistics on disease prevalence compete with a success story like that?

In addition to giving testimony to the effectiveness of advertising, and to the failure of methods that just present the awful facts, I think part of the reason that statistics can't compete with pretty girls drinking soda pop is that, however indisputable, numbers and graphs can be off-putting. I can tell you that my own eyes glaze over at the first mention 37.8 percent or, ".... increasing by 6.7 percent per year".

I talked about facing up to the fact that we are all going to die. But I didn't do it to demoralize you into resigned surrender. In this book, I offer positive strategies to change your focus away from that gloomy prospect. With a doctor's ancient dictum, primum non nocerum (First do no harm) firmly in mind, I instead, take an approach of hope and encouragement, based on knowledge and understanding—specifically, yours. If not yours now, then that which will be yours when you've finished reading this book.

That said, I am going to assume that the last thing you want to do is to read a text on biochemistry or physiology. So I will try to keep it as simple as fits the immediate need to understand the point. In professional quarters, this may garner me accusations of over-simplifying, but so what? If this book can guide even a few diabetics into a longer, healthier, more satisfying life, it will be well worth the effort.

As we go along, you might find me writing "carbs" for carbohydrates and "sugar" for blood glucose. I'll talk about "plasma" glucose, too. It's the same as blood glucose. Plasma just designates the colorless liquid portion of all the stuff, liquid and solid, that flows through our blood vessels.

This is not a diet book. It won't show you how to lose eight pounds in two weeks, or get into that bikini that you bought last winter. There are only a few illustrative recipes. But there is much information on how to *think* about food, and its correlative, the nourishment it is supposed to provide. If all you want to do is lose enough weight to fit into that bikini this summer, buy some other book. Because unless you have a will of iron, whatever weight you lose on such diets is almost guaranteed to come back with a vengeance. And let's face it. If you did have that kind of self-discipline, you wouldn't have a weight problem to begin with, would you?

My strategy is to help you break the vicious cycle of bad habits by motivating you to make a complete life-style change, and by giving you the understanding and the psychological tools that will help make the change permanent. In the process, I'll show you some frequently-overlooked but surprisingly effective methods that you can put to use.

If you have Type II diabetes, or have been told you are pre-diabetic, and are worried about what happens to you if or when you get it, this book is for you. If you have a weight problem and a family history of diabetes, this book is for you. It can also help if you have only a moderate weight problem and don't like what you see in the mirror. I must warn that it pulls no punches. There are some hard truths here. But there are solutions too. And in the final analysis, truth is always kinder than the lies we tell ourselves to avoid it.

2

My Own Discovery

In the late spring of 2000, my last year of medical practice before retirement, I went for my hospital reappointment physical exam, an annual event for attending doctors at our hospital. Bloods were drawn as we say, and the doctor did the usual ECG, poked me here and there, listened to my heart, and ordered a chest x-ray, and urine analysis.

In due course, the blood chemistry results came back, including the two-hour post-prandial blood glucose (Two hours after a meal). If you are not familiar with this particular test, it is a blood sample to measure plasma glucose that is drawn two hours after an ordinary meal. It is the best simple indicator that something might be amiss. It is far and away the single most useful test for patients already diagnosed with diabetes, and for people who are diabetes suspects (more about this later).

Well, among the long list of normal results, I was astonished to see a blood sugar of 238. Normal plasma glucose ranges from 85 to 110 or so, depending on when food was taken, and in a healthy individual, is very well controlled between those two levels.

The test results were a mistake, of course. Somebody had mislabeled the tubes of blood. *Well,* I thought. *We'll just see about that.*

Sometime during the following week, I wrote myself a lab request for another two-hour post-prandial blood glucose, and on the day of the test went out and had a cheeseburger, a shake, and a slice of apple pie for lunch, before heading over to the hospital lab. In the days before the glucose tolerance test was introduced, doctors might ask a patient to have a breakfast or lunch that included a sugar load—say a milk shake or an ice cream sundae, then two hours later, blood for a plasma-glucose would be drawn to see how the patient handled such a sugar load. That's what I was doing. Since the introduction of the glucose tolerance test, a laboratory-controlled evaluation that provides much more information, doctors don't get to please their patients with instructions to eat ice cream sundaes and the like.

The hospital lab technician laughed when I told her of my suspicions about erroneously labeled tubes.

"With all the malpractice suits?" she said. "We've pretty much nailed that one. The chance of mixing up blood sample tubes is very slim. Your response to the first test is typical though, especially among our doctors. You all think you're armor-plated."

At that time, my body weight, on a smallish, 5-foot 11-inch frame, was two-hundred pounds, give or take four or five pounds heavier or lighter depending on the season and whether I felt hungry as I walked past a pizzeria in mid-afternoon. My work kept me so busy that I didn't have time to worry about what I was putting into my stomach. At least that's what I told myself. I wasn't quite a couch potato, but I was well on my way toward what might be called an "office" potato. Even so, I spent my days lecturing patients about the evils of eating too much food and exercising too little.

"Don't do as I do, do as I say," I rationalized. Naturally, the rules didn't apply for me. The lab technician was right. Like all doctors, I was impervious. What was her expression? Armor-plated? The common-sense rules of a healthy life-style didn't apply.

But each succeeding generation of my suits, sport

jackets, and dress shirts, was larger. Over the years, my waist grew to forty inches, then to forty-two inches. I gave my outgrown clothes to the local chapter of the Salvation Army. I was comforted by the knowledge that I was helping the needy.

Then, after my little come-uppance at the hands of the lab technician (who was herself at least eighty pounds overweight), reality struck, with its familiar hard blow. The second two-hour post-prandial blood sugar was 216. Now I understood why earlier that spring, when I had had some benign skin lesions excised, the incisions were extremely slow to heal (one of the problems of diabetes). I called a doctor friend to schedule a work up. He said,

"Work up? Work up for what? Nothing serious, I hope. Not an old campaigner like you." (Like most of us, he was infected with the impervious-bug too.)

"Diabetes," I said. "My plasma glucose was 238 at my hospital re-appointment exam." I could almost hear Allen cringing over the phone. He said, "Ouch!"

The Diabetic Workup

From the patient's point of view, the work-up for diabetes isn't complicated, or difficult to understand. A good history-of-present-illness (HPI), a general physical exam, a dilated eye exam to detect any diabetic changes in the retina and to check for cataracts and glaucoma—conditions that are more common in diabetics—and the usual lab work, including a complete blood count, a urine analysis, and some other tests particular to diabetes, are usually sufficient. I've mentioned one of them before, the *glucose tolerance test*, in which a fasting patient (that means nothing by mouth since midnight or approximately eight hours) has an initial blood sample drawn as a baseline, then is given a fizzy orange drink containing either 75 or 100 grams of glucose. Blood samples are then drawn every half-hour for two hours, and a final sample is drawn at the end of three hours.

As you might imagine, the resultant blood sugar measurements can be reported as a list of figures, or they can be plotted on a graph. Over the three hours' time, the plasma glucose rises in response to the dietary sugar load entering the bloodstream. Then, some time along the way, the number starts to fall again, as an outpouring of insulin from the pancreatic beta cells kicks in to normalize the elevated blood sugar. How high the sugar goes, how fast it rises, and how long it stays up before coming down to normal again, helps the doctor determine how your system handles a sugar load, and helps him determine whether or not you have diabetes.

The other test, often done at the same time, is a hemoglobin A-1-C test, or Hgb A1C test. It is also marvelously useful. With a tube of venous blood, the doctor can determine whether a patient's plasma glucose has been elevated over the previous four to six weeks, not when, or for how long, but just that the blood sugar was elevated for some period of time. The result is reported as a percentage. In our lab, anything below 6.5 percent is in the normal range.

> *The HGB A1C test measures the percentage of red blood cells that have blood glucose attached, (or bound) to them. The RBCs that have glucose linked to them are said to be glycated. In a non-diabetic person, this is about 5 percent of the circulating RBCs. It means that about 5 in every 100 red blood cells are glycated. In a diabetic, the percentage is generally much higher, and can be as high as 25% when glucose levels are out of control for a long period of time. The more glucose floating around in the circulating blood, the more it links up with (glycates) the red blood cells.*
>
> *The Hgb A1C test is accurate to within about a half of one percent, depending on the lab. (Pretty useful test!)*

When all the results were in, I got a phone call.

"Well," the doctor said, "I guess we've made a diagnosis. Common things occur most commonly, right? The good news is, it's not bad. There's a good chance that you'll be able to control it with diet and weight loss."

"I'm a jump ahead, Allen. I've already put myself on a diet. *Very* low carbohydrate, and no dietary sugar. Zero. I've never had a sweet-tooth, so that will be the easiest part."

"Well," he said, "It sounds a little extreme, but okay. See me in six months and we'll re-check things. And don't forget the other half of the equation."

I knew exactly what he meant. Exercise.

But that part of it didn't happen. If it had, I probably would have less reason to write this book. Can I say that again? *If I had combined exercise with my diet, I very likely would not have had to write this book.* (Would it be too cheeky of me to suggest that if you had placed yourself on an effective exercise program back when, you probably would not now be having to read this book?)

I wonder how many of the twenty-six million-or-so Americans with discovered or undiscovered Type II diabetes, realize the significance of what I just said. Because, while I managed the sugar problem very well by dieting, I initially completely neglected my doctor's "other half of the equation". And, for a lot of reasons, many of which we will explore in this book, neglecting that half of the equation is what gets most diabetics into trouble.

I know. You're going to say, "Oh, come on, Doc. You mean to say that the secret to controlling my sugar is as simple as exercising?"

The short answer is, "Almost." I'll talk about diet and weight loss too, but I want to go on record here and now, by telling you that exercise is so important that it has a more beneficial effect on the control of adult-onset diabetes than diet does. This is not to say that if you exercise, dietary considerations can or should be de-emphasized, or ignored. It's just that contrary to what seems to be generally accepted as effective diabetes therapy, diet alone is not enough, not even when coupled with medicine. As you will learn in this book, adding exercise into the mix can change your life in ways you never would have imagined.

Unfortunately, the exercise portion is so often neglected, that the majority of diabetics doom themselves to early, completely unnecessary diabetic complications. It doesn't matter whether you're forty or seventy-five, or what kind of shape you're in, good, terrible, or not so terrible, there's an exercise regimen, probably very simple, that will improve your health, increase your energy level, improve your mental clarity and your longevity, to say nothing of your happiness quotient. Depending on your weight, age and present physical condition, your exercise commitment might commence with a half-mile walk, or with walking around the dining room table ten times a day. And I'm not going to leave it at that. As we go along, I will explain exactly which types of exercise are best, how to do them, what they will accomplish for you, and the precautions associated with them.

Chapter summary: Things to think about

Normal blood sugar levels: 85 to 110 on your
finger-stick glucose meter, depending on time of
last food intake

The 'at-home' two-hour post-prandial blood sugar is a
finger-stick blood-sugar measurement 2 hours after a
meal—the only really useful at-home test.

Glucose tolerance test measures how well your body
handles a sugar load.

Simple diabetic work-up: history and general physical
exam, dilated eye exam, complete blood count (CBC),
fasting blood sugar, hemoglobin A1C tests, and
glucose tolerance test.

Hemoglobin A1C test can reveal whether your blood
sugar has been elevated for a significant length of
time over the past 4 to 6 weeks; informative and
useful.

The super-important other half of the equation—
exercise.

3

The Usual, and wrong approach.

And the Fix.

Knowing the facts as well as I did, and deciding not to get started exercising at once, I should have been kicked in the you-know-what. But here's the way my thinking went (I'm sure that you too have a little story you could tell).

I knew that if I curtailed my carbohydrate intake severely enough I would lose lots of weight, so I told myself that for the time being there was good enough reason to defer exercising. I was looking forward to retiring from medical practice the following winter, and I was busier than ever. Sure, in spare moments, I pictured myself riding bikes, jogging, lifting weights, swimming at the club, looking fit. The usual empty dreams of glory. But the simple truth—and it's probably true for you as well, if you're anything like me —is that although my body could pretty much do anything I asked of it, I hadn't exercised in a regular, programmed way during the forty years of my working life.

Why did I think that retiring would change my habits? It's not that I wasn't active. I was, but only insofar as I needed to be to do the things a reasonably active life requires. In short, I never *deliberately* worked up a sweat.

Instead, like most non-exercisers, I rationalized. It's so much easier to rationalize than it is to face hard facts, and to do something about them. *In case you've forgotten, rationalize means ". . to devise self-satisfying but incorrect reasons for one's behavior".*

I thought, "I'll just concentrate on getting skinny. Then I'll feel so much better that I'll *want* to get going. Besides, I walk a lot, and always have. That's a start. And every little bit helps, right?"

And it's true. Every little bit does help, and when you're thin you do feel better. You want to be active. You want to exercise. And I did too—a little. But only a little.

As I thinned down, I started to walk more. To improve my balance, and strengthen my calf muscles, I stood on one leg while brushing my teeth or talking on the phone. I never sat down to pull on my trousers. I hoisted my wife's three-pound dumbbells while we watched TV. I made it a point to take stairs whenever I could, and I shunned escalators. I parked my car farther away. Over the months, one or two flights of stairs became easy. My weight was dropping. So far, so good, I reasoned.

Exercise and Diabetes

There's only one thing wrong with this picture. And this is where you come in. Because chances are, you're just like I am.

If you want to live a long life, it's not enough to ride a bike on weekends, go to the gym once or twice a week, play a round of golf or lift dumbbells while you watch TV with your significant other.

This pretend approach goes to the very heart of why we Americans are experiencing an obesity and diabetes epidemic. We do a little exercise, either on purpose or by accident, going to the gym occasionally, or playing a leisurely round of golf, and we rationalize (there's that word again) that we lead an active life style. Part of the reason is that physical activity makes us feel good about ourselves, and infuses us with hope. But unless it becomes a regular part of our everyday life, it won't fulfill its promise, but instead will give us false confidence.

To be beneficial, an exercise program must start out as a program. It must be regular, progressive, and if possible, supervised. At least until it becomes so much a part of you that you know the routine like the back of your hand, and if you skip a day you will sense that something is wrong, something is missing. Otherwise it will just be doing it occasionally, feeling good about having done it, vowing to continue, breaking our vow the first time it is inconvenient, and gradually losing interest and stopping altogether.

It takes some months to build regular exercise into a habit, and it is vitally important to continue the program long enough to establish that habit, to make certain that it is a part of you, and not just an "add-on" that can be abandoned with little or no regret.

If you decide to attend a gym and engage a trainer on a once or twice-a-week basis, it's actually easier if you do not make a concerted effort to learn and memorize the individual parts of the workout—the individual warming up exercises and stretches, the work-out patterns, and the cooling down stretches. Let the trainer do the thinking. Allow him to guide you through it, session after session, week after week, until your program becomes second nature. The only thing you have to concentrate on, is getting yourself into the groove, doing those allotted count-down minutes on the stationary bike or the treadmill, doing those reps, letting worries and external stimuli slip away as you communicate with your body.

Aren't humans incredible? We manage somehow to separate our minds from our bodies, effectively living our lives inside of our heads, as though our bodies aren't even attached to us. In fact, this ability is one of the root causes of obesity; our formidable mental skills allow us to

> *imagine, and even come to believe ourselves to be other than we really are. William Shakespeare had an explanation, and hidden in it is the remedy.*
>
> *He had Hamlet say, ". . . for use can change the very stamp of nature."*
>
> *What he meant was, if you act like you want to be, you will actually come to be the way you act. The theory, proved by practice, is to think like an active person, and act like an active person, this means actually physically doing it, and feeling that it's the way you are, down inside, and you will actually become an active, fitter person.*

After a few weeks of learning the exercise routine, you will automatically begin to anticipate, to know, what your trainer is going to select as the next warm-up stretch or exercise. This is when the process will almost have become an ingrained habit, a satisfying part of your week that you will look forward to with pleasure.

For those who absolutely, positively cannot access a professional trainer in a gym, even on a once-a-week basis, the back of this book contains a program with built-in safeguards, and a schedule that will help you get started. I must warn however, that when it comes to sweating it out in your own rec-room or bedroom, it takes a lot of self-discipline—more than most of us have. Let's face it. If we had the kind of discipline it takes to develop and stick to an exercise program on our own, we very likely wouldn't have gotten into trouble in the first place. You wouldn't be reading this book, and very likely I would not have written it.

But please don't come down on yourself too hard. You have lots and lots of company. That said though, do give it a little objective analysis. Don't let the "everybody does it" cop-out provide an excuse. This is one time when twenty million Frenchmen, or a hundred million Americans, *can* be wrong. Not including children, that's how many American adults are *significantly* overweight. A hundred million!

In addition to this seriously overweight group, the most recent figures state that an unbelievable sixty-five percent of Americans are *moderately* overweight, weighing in at 30-or-more pounds above normal. We are nearly 300 million people. What is 65 percent of that number? Would you believe that 200 million people in the United States are either slightly, moderately or seriously overweight? So it's easy to see that the "everybody does it" rationalization seems to be batting nearly a thousand here. And more importantly, within those numbers, lies the reason why you shouldn't fall for it.

What's so Important About Exercise?

One of the reasons that I believe in, and emphasize the importance of exercise is that nearly two-thirds of diabetics do not die from their disease. We die from something else— something preventable for most of us, at least throughout what should be the best of our so-called golden years. We die from heart trouble. And stroke. I said I wasn't going to depress you with numbers and percentages, but just this once I'm giving myself a pass. Because I know how to change the numbers for you.

Change your mind—and your life

Traditionally, most newly-diagnosed diabetics are told that in order to control blood sugar, diet is of first importance. In my opinion it is not. Controlling blood cholesterol with exercise (and with statins, if necessary) to assure that the sugar you eat gets burned as energy, and not stored as fat, is far more important to a long life. As you will learn in the chapters ahead, regular exercise lowers cholesterol, reduces body weight, lowers blood sugar, and raises our energy level. The emphasis here is on "regular".

I hope to show you why and how to do it; how to keep your weight down, have plenty of energy, become stronger as you get older, or at least hold your own, and reduce your medicines to an absolute minimum, possibly cut them out entirely if you have only an early intolerance to glucose and not already well-established type II diabetes.

Do you like that possibility? Why *wouldn't* you?

I don't care how old, or how young you are now, or in what physical condition you are at present, you can be much better. With a body that within reasonable limits, will do your will without protesting, and a clear mind to supervise it. If I can change the way you see yourself, clear your mind of popular misconceptions about food, and convince you to think about nourishment and physical activity in a new way, changing the size and shape of your body will be the easy part.

Chapter Summary; Things to think about.

Concentrating on diet, the usual—and wrong approach.

Every little bit helps; walking more, taking stairs instead of escalators, parking farther away, lifting dumbbells while watching TV. But by themselves, they are not enough.

Exercise must be regular, progressive, and programmatic.

Improve your balance; stand on one leg whenever possible (when you're on the phone, while brushing your teeth, washing your hands, etc. Think of some yourself.)

Exercise: the surest way to prevent heart disease and stroke.

Rationalization; how it hurts.

The Real Secret: change you mind—and Your life cholesterol is of great importance for diabetics.

Exercise lowers cholesterol better than diet does and helps stabilize blood sugar levels and reduces blood-sugar spikes. And it's easier than you think.

4

Diet, Calories, Carbohydrates

But first things first. I want to tell you some more of my own story, reasoning flaws and all, because it's probably a lot like yours. We'll deal with the cholesterol problem later, when I can give it full measure. Considering that it's what tries to kill us all, and still now in the twenty-first century, is better at it than any other single cause, if we're going to make an attempt to lick it, it deserves a chapter or two of its own.

When I got the lab test results back, I took a really good look at myself in the mirror after work one day. I saw a naked, pear-shaped, middle-aged man holding a sheaf of lab results. "Face it," I said to the mirror. "You've become a fat man."

Despite my admonitions about exercise, you'll soon see that like you, and probably your doctor as well, I began by thinking, "diet, diet, diet!" So the first thing I did was ask myself the wrong question. If I want to lose weight, I thought, what can I eat and in what quantities? And what shouldn't I eat? Believe it or not, they are the wrong questions!

And since we are presumably facing facts in this book, we should admit too that no matter how necessary, how central it is to successful diabetes control, your exercise program alone will not be the entire armamentarium against diabetes and coronary artery disease. There is no magic bullet, only honest, thoughtful analysis of the problem, coupled with a willingness to do what's necessary to beat it.

So I'm going to talk about diet first. If only because that's the way I approached it, and I want you to see the flaws in my reasoning so you don't waste two or three years of your life thinking that diet is the be-all end-all, and ending up with a coronary artery stent like I did. So I want to take you through it from the beginning. Because buried among the bad decisions are pearls of dietary wisdom. You'll need them too. I said exercise is paramount. I didn't say it was everything, or that nothing else counts.

Calories or Carbohydrates?

Instead of keeping track of my caloric intake, I chose to start by counting carbohydrates. There's a good reason that I did. Compared to counting calories—375 here, 750 there—keeping track of carbohydrates is a snap, and in the end, amounts to the same thing, a way of counting the ingestion of calories and starches. Isn't it easier to think about limiting your intake to say, 50 or 60 grams of carbohydrates a day, than to do the arithmetic for 1,850 calories? Or 2,200 calories? No contest. And of course, reducing carbohydrates automatically reduces caloric intake.

And here's a point that that is often overlooked. Reducing carbohydrates lowers your intake of an entire food group that is fattening—all the starches, sweet and not sweet. Doesn't concentrating on calories instead do the same thing? Because of psychology, not quite. When we count calories we tend to concentrate our calorie-lowering efforts on the sugars that are sweet. I learned that in my medical practice. It's natural to mentally associate calories with sweet-tasting foods. The trouble is, we tend to gloss over the rest of the foods that pile on the pounds. If you count carbohydrates, it simplifies your life, and it accomplishes the same thing a little more efficiently—it helps reduce your intake of *all* fattening foods.

Like caloric content, carbohydrates are listed on every package of prepared foods; on canned soups, broths, and vegetables, all frozen foods, packaged dry foods of all kinds. It is only missing on fresh fruits and vegetables, and what I call "loose" snacks; bagels, scoops of ice cream, Danish pastry and the like. But when I decided to cut my carbohydrate intake to the bone, it didn't take a dietitian (or a cardiologist) to tell me that as well as avoiding ice cream, pretzels and potato chips are also out; too much hidden sugar and are too high in saturated fat and trans-fatty acids (don't forget the underlying diagnosis here).

People ask me if I had put myself on the "Atkins" diet. No, I didn't. Nor was it any other pre-packaged, formulaic diet plan "as endorsed by," (. . . .fill in the celebrity doctor's name). My counting carbohydrates instead of calories was not *eliminating* carbohydrates, which was the concept that the original Atkins diet seemed to hang its hat on. I just decided to count carbohydrates instead of calories because they're easier to keep track of, and for the other reasons mentioned above, and then striving to lower their presence in my diet sufficient to lose weight. But in my enthusiasm engendered by the rapid results, I went overboard. I reduced my carbohydrate intake to almost nil, and paid the price by clogging my coronary arteries via food replacements that were inappropriate for my sedentary life style.

It is important to understand that I am not suggesting that the quantity of calories in the diet is unimportant. When it comes to reducing body weight, calories are a pivotal element. But as any failed dieter will verify, trying to lose weight by counting calories is a difficult, thankless task, and we have now come to understand, is more often than not actually counter-productive when it comes to losing weight permanently. As we go along, I will explain the reasons, one of which has elements in it similar to the fallacy of trying to quit smoking by "cutting down". It never works because it can't work. Teasing ourselves with small doses of the indulgence that got us where we are will never rid us of the desire. Think about it. It just prolongs the agony, doesn't it? And the other thing is, that although they lower their overall number, calorie-counters usually continue to include the same sweet foods in their diets, reducing, but not eliminating them from their diets, as I stated above. Later on I'll discuss how sugar actually conditions our taste buds to want more, and what effect that has on our food choices.

Food for Thought

So in reducing carbohydrate intake, our aim is not to eliminate carbohydrates from the diet, only to lower the quantity we are ingesting, and in that way, lower our caloric intake automatically. In choosing foods for the carbohydrate side of our diet, it is important to select quality carbohydrates; whole grains, vegetables, certain legumes, and (some) fruits, which are more slowly digested than processed foods, and other sources of sweet, empty calories in processed foods. Quality carbohydrates raise blood sugar more slowly. Also, they do not tickle our "sweet tooth" as much, and that lessens our urge for sweets. I'll talk a lot more about this later on too. It's an important key in the process of switching to healthier foods.

But even among low-carbohydrate foods, we must exercise care in our choices. Many foods contain zero, or near-zero carbohydrates, and relatively few calories, and are attractive to the dieter because of it; red meats, poultry, fresh and canned fish, cheeses, eggs, and many prepared meat products such as hamburger, frankfurters, sausages, packaged pork and beef products, and lunch meats. My understanding of this contributed to my first big mistake, because while these choices have few or no carbohydrates, most are high in saturated fat and trans fats and are very dangerous because of it.

That is my objection to the original Atkins diet, especially when it is not supervised by a doctor or nutritionist, and combined with a rigorous exercise program. Recently, the sponsors of the program have recognized this lapse, and are busy correcting it, but recent studies are not encouraging as regards the incidence heart attack and stroke among Atkins-plan dieters.

About quantities; the National Academy of Sciences recommends that the minimum amount of carbohydrate needed to stay healthy is 130 grams a day. To my mind, this is a dangerously irresponsible recommendation. Among all the nourishing, low-carbohydrate and low calorie foods available to us on this wonderful planet, choosing to ingest one hundred and thirty grams of carbohydrates every day is one of the surest ways to slide into obesity and the degenerative diseases that go with it.

Get in the habit of reading ingredients labels. Check the size of the serving at the top, then the amount and types of fats that that portion contains, along with its sugars, carbohydrates, calories, and sodium. Below the nutritional values there is an ingredients-list, where ingredients are listed in the order of their amounts. The main ingredients are at the top. Those in lesser proportion follow according to their quantities. And at the end, the additives, food colors, and preservatives are listed, because they are present in the smallest quantities. My rule on these ingredients is, with very occasional exceptions, if you cannot pronounce it, don't eat it.

Here are some food exchanges that are not often mentioned, but are probably more important to long life than any bread exchange you could make. Make up your mind today, starting right now, to give up bacon, processed lunch meats and pork products, hamburger made from beef, lamb, steaks and chops. Start by simply not buying them at the market. Think about this; *If you don't take it home you won't eat it.*

Because of the diabetic's propensity toward heart disease, fats are every bit as dangerous as sugar. For hamburger, think ground turkey breast instead. There's even a low-fat variety with 3% fat content, as opposed to regular ground turkey, which has 7%. Instead of steaks and chops, plan meals around fish. Salmon burgers are wonderful. Make vegetables a large part of your meals, especially the cruciferous ones. They will help save your life.

Replace the chops and steaks with fish, ground turkey or chicken, skinless chicken from which you have trimmed visible fat, egg whites, tofu, and fat-free cheeses. It is possible to give up chops roasts and steaks entirely, and still eat a nourishing diet. And fill the rest of your plate with cruciferous vegetables and greens. With the exception of pumpkin, zucchini, and squash, be careful with limas, peas, corn, and other starchy vegetables.

Difficult? If it were easy we wouldn't be sick. But for me, there's no contest between having a healthier, longer life, and the temporary satisfaction of a stomach full of fatty foods and the shortened life that goes with that kind of diet. In the food section of this book, I will tell you how to eat and enjoy chicken and turkey without having to worry too much about its fat content.

Chapter summary: Things to think about:

Diet is simply not enough. We must include my doctor's "other half".... exercise.

Count carbohydrates instead of calories. They're easier to keep track of and it will make you think of the entire range of starchy foods instead of just the obviously sugary ones.

Low carbohydrates means low calories.

Quality carbs are important. They help reduce spikes in blood sugar. Slower digestion is the reason.

Don't aim for zero carbs like I did; without a really rigorous exercise program and a doctor's help it's far too dangerous.

Question the veracity of everything you read about food and nutrition, even when the source seems impeccable. Sometimes even the experts get it wrong.

Read the small print on labels; ingredients are always listed in the order of their presence. If you see a lot of stuff you can't pronounce, don't eat it.

5

Free Foods

There are some other foods I should have included in my first low-carb crash diet but didn't. These are so low in calories and carbohydrates, and otherwise so good for us, that when considering them for a diabetic or weight-losing diet it is usually unnecessary to count their carbohydrate or calorie content at all. Hence the name, "free" foods, a term that has been around for awhile without attracting much notice, which is unfortunate because free foods are of tremendous help in the battles against high blood sugar and excessive body weight (to say nothing of heart disease and stroke).

Free foods are low in sugar, generally very low in calories and fat, and are usually eaten in small quantities to assuage hunger. Because they are nourishing, and do not significantly raise blood sugar, they can also be eaten in quantities sufficient for a light lunch or dinner. There is an extensive list of free foods in Chapter Eleven where I discuss their use and value in depth.

Of course the diabetic eye always darts down the nutrients list to the sugars. Almost all foods contain sugar. In the real world, it is impossible to avoid. I noticed that a can of soda contains about thirty-five grams of sugar. That's nearly half of the amount that the technician gives you in the glucose tolerance test (usually 75 grams), a test that challenges your body's sugar-handling system to find out whether or not you have diabetes. How many sodas does the average teen-ager put away in a day's time? Scary.

I recently saw an article in a local newspaper that suggested that mothers instruct their children to drink diet soda instead of regular soda, but not more than four cans a day because the long-term health effects of artificial sweeteners are not fully understood. *Four cans of artificially-sweetened soda a day?* Food colorings? Brand-specific, "secret formula" chemicals? Artificial sweeteners, whose long-term health effects are largely unknown, and have recently been shown to place steady diet-soda drinkers at risk for type II diabetes just like real sugar does? And which contain phosphoric acid to leach the calcium out of our bones, and condition our taste buds to want more sweets the same way sugar does? All I have to say is, Wow!

Toppling An Icon

One of the aims of a diet of course, is to limit our caloric intake, and contrary to the thrust of nearly every advertised diet plan, that's more effectively accomplished by choosing *what* we eat rather than concentrating on *how much.* Many diet-plan managers seem to be so homed in on curtailing portions and adjusting the calorie-content of otherwise-unacceptable food choices, that they miss this point completely.

Of course limiting portions is one way to approach it. But it's not the only way, nor is it anywhere near the best way in my opinion. I touched on this topic in the chapter above. If you need proof, see the dozens of diet plans out there in television land. Do any of them really work? Are users actually losing weight *and keeping it off?* Take a look at the diet-book section in your local book store. It's probably ten feet long, and two shelves deep. Many plans are full of promises that if you follow their instructions, you will lose eight or ten pounds in two or three weeks. Sure you will, but what happens after that? How do you change your life so that the new you will last a lifetime, and not just for the rest of the summer, or until the wedding is over?

This is an important concept to understand, for it is the essential difference between quick weight loss which is physiologically suspect (and almost never lasts), and permanent re-shaping of your body, accompanied by improved control of blood sugar levels by the principles outlined in this book.

Quality versus Quantity

The other day at a department store lunch room, just as I finished a portion of baked salmon and a mélange of mixed vegetables that included zucchini, egg plant, tomato, onion and peppers, an overweight lady in her late thirties sat down opposite me. On her plate were Swedish meatballs in brown gravy and two boiled potatoes with parsley and butter on them. For her dessert she had a generous wedge of chocolate cake with icing—to go with her can of soda. I was sorry to see that her thighs were so fat that she was already beginning to waddle as she walked.

It was obvious that she hadn't discovered the secret. A secret that is as simple as broccoli versus bread, fish versus Swedish meatballs, tea versus soda water—*what instead of how much*. It helps us rid ourselves of the taste memory of sweets and fats that those foods imbed into our taste buds, and that is one of the real secrets to successful dieting. It takes time and persistence, but the goal is well worth it. I will discuss this more fully in succeeding chapters, and suggest simple ways to accomplish it.

I think having to limit yourself to one or two slices of "American" white or whole wheat bread per day, or using it as an exchange food for some other starchy no-no, is just too sad. It keeps bread in your mind as a food choice when it should be long gone, and it exactly illustrates what this book is about.

"But Doctor," you say. "I need my bread! Even if it's only a slice or two." Yes, I know. You've been eating bread all of your life. I have too. And I too love it. But ask yourself what you would rather do, coddle your bread-habit straight into an early grave, or stay alive, and looking forward to each new day for many more years? Alive to see beautiful sunsets, to taste fresh air, to love someone dear, to hug the grandkids, to experience winter and spring, and rain, and starry skies, a full moon climbing the evening sky?

That's exactly the choice, isn't it? And is it really a choice? Not for me. I refuse to pin my life and my existence on this earth to a slice of bread, or cake, or a plate of pasta. If the man said to me, "You've abused your body to the point where you've seriously compromised your life-expectancy. If you want twenty more years instead of an early death, it's broccoli and spring water and nothing else!" I'd head for the vegetable bin without a whimper. Isn't that in a sense, exactly what our diabetes, or our thunder thighs are telling us? "Lose it or else" is one of the unspoken messages we ought to be receiving.

Chapter summary: Things to think about

In this chapter; a brief introduction to free foods and why they're good for us

Soda Water—its prevalence and its dangers; whether regular or artificially sweetened

Think about quality versus quantity; explore the concept.

How much we eat is not nearly as important as what we eat—broccoli versus bread.

Don't exchange potato for bread, exchange it for green vegetables. Then forget the bread.

Don't give your taste buds bad memories with sweet-tasting treats.

Don't trade your life for the temporary pleasure of something good to eat!

6

"Losing weight is easy"

I said counting carbohydrates is easier than counting calories, but I didn't say what you've perhaps already guessed—or knew. That as far as the bloodstream is concerned, carbohydrates *are* calories. And sweet or not, they are also sugars. Because they are digested at a slower rate, complex carbohydrates do not cause as rapid an elevation, or "spike" in blood sugar, as simple sugars do, and that is why they are promoted as being healthier for us. This spike, or rapid elevation of blood sugar, that occurs soon after eating easily digested sweets, causes an outpouring of insulin, which can lower blood sugar to below-normal levels, triggering a second hunger—the old Chinese dinner syndrome. You remember; you're hungry again in two hours. It is also involved in the "I suffer from low blood sugar" condition people complain of, a condition we won't deal with in this book, because although it can be a sign of undiagnosed or incorrectly-treated diabetes, it also has several other causes unrelated to the problems we're trying to solve in this book.

Complex Carbohydrates

Although it takes longer to digest whole grains, pasta, potatoes, certain whole grain breakfast cereals, and other non-sweet starches, along with the B vitamins, the sugars they contain still get absorbed into the blood stream. I'm not convinced that the advantage of slow absorption outweighs the disadvantage of pumping in a carbohydrate load of the magnitude that even these "good" carbohydrates provide.

I guess that with the logic that a step in the right direction is better than no step at all, many popular diet plans suggest complex carbohydrates as a substitute for other, more harmful sugars contained in pastries, ice cream and the like. A well-intentioned idea to be sure, but the downside is the false comfort they provide. As in, "I'll eat these "good" complex carbs instead of the sweet stuff and I'll be safe. And hey—since they're *good* carbs, I can really chow down!"

A case in point; the federal government is now beginning to admit that its much-publicized food pyramid—the one which emphasizes daily consumption of several portions of complex carbohydrates—may have been designed to help grain farmers find a larger market for their crops—an amazingly brazen deception by our Washington "leaders". And isn't it interesting that *our* food pyramid is strikingly similar to the one that is employed in stockyards to fatten cattle for market? Not including third world people, the vast majority of today's workers are not shoveling concrete for a living, or felling trees. We're sitting at desks of course, or standing behind counters. Acknowledgment of this is evidenced by the fact that because of our sedentary lifestyles, many of our larger apartment houses provide treadmills and stationary bikes right in the building in gyms set aside for the purpose. And the federal government has recently announced a new food pyramid with re-arranged priorities.

Sugars - what makes them sweet? And why you should know about them

The information that follows is not complicated, and it's useful, because it helps you understand the different rates of digestion of the various sugars and starches. And that makes a difference in how high and how fast your blood sugar rises after ingesting them.

The essential difference between sugar-bowl sugar and complex carbohydrates like pasta, rice, potato and bread, is that *sucrose* (table sugar) is a quickly digested compound of just two molecules chemically fastened together. It is called a disaccharide. ("di" means "two", or "a pair").

Complex carbohydrates on the other hand, are longer chains of sugar molecules. They are called polysaccharides. The longer the chain, the less sweet they are; table sugar, honey, and maple syrup are short chain sugars and are sweet tasting. Pasta and rice? A whole gang of sugar molecules hooked together in a long chain—not sweet. Do you want me to show you their formulas? I think not. You didn't buy this book to study chemistry. It's a waste of your time and it's beside the point.

But what isn't beside the point is the little-known (or inadequately-publicized) fact that I briefly mentioned above. In the process of digestion, *all* carbohydrates, long chain, intermediate chain or short chain, are broken down to simple sugar before they can be transported across the intestinal wall into the blood stream. The only real difference to you is in how easily and how fast each is digested, and whether you will have a resultant quick high spike in the blood glucose, or only a slow rise.

The significance to diabetics is obvious and important. It means that no matter how we euphemize it, what we call it, or whether or not it tastes sweet, if it's a starch food— French fries, pancakes, bread, packaged breakfast cereal, rice, macaroni, fruit, ice cream or wedding cake—the carbohydrate part of it (and of course the sweet, simple sugar part of it as well) enters and circulates in the

bloodstream essentially as glucose. That is to say, *as sugar.*
Along with giving some thought to how rapidly and how
high various starches and sugars raise the blood glucose,
that's what I want you to take out of this; table sugar, pasta,
rice, potato, bread, all enter the blood stream as glucose.
The only difference is in how fast they are altered in the
intestine and transported into the blood stream.

Wrong Choices

Well, where does that leave us? We can't eat sugar, we
can't eat carbohydrates. What's left, you ask. When I
discovered I had diabetes, I asked myself exactly that
question. Take away starches and sugars and what's left in
the diabetes larder? Proteins and fats, and green vegetables
(cruciferous and leafy).

That week when I got that look at myself in the mirror,
that really good look I mentioned above, I decided to go
food shopping with my wife to see if I could find some
foods with no carbs at all. Another big mistake. I came home
with thirty-five dollars worth of cheeses, canned tuna,
canned salmon, herring and sardines, cartons of egg whites,
whole eggs, jars of pickles, cucumbers, peanuts in the shell
(more about peanuts anon), chicken breasts ground and
whole, ditto turkey, hot dogs and lunch meats, and salmon
fillets for the charcoal grill. Nary a carb in sight!

But was my carbohydrate-free diet like the then-popular
Atkins diet? Not quite, because I included lots of green
vegetables cold and hot, I substituted egg whites for whole
eggs (most mornings) and I ate fresh fish two or three times
a week. My S.O. is a great Italian cook, and saw to it that I
got generous amounts of cooked and raw greens nearly
every day—escarole, spinach, kale, rob broccoli—even turnip
greens, which are surprisingly tasty. I must admit though,
that meat was a mainstay—pork tenderloins, the occasional
steak, lots of chicken and turkey. I gave up the frankfurters
early on. Without the roll and tasty, sugary ketchup they're
just too chemically-awful as a steady part of anybody's diet.

It was going to be my brave new world. My breakfast, previously oatmeal or shredded wheat, or maybe a buttered bagel or toast, would now be an omelet of eggs or commercially-prepared egg whites. With one change—no bread, rolls, or bagels.

Breakfast carbohydrates? I counted them—fewer than ten. Lunch, previously a slice of pizza (or two), was now tuna salad or an individual-size can of salmon with lemon juice. Another thirty grams of carbohydrates *not* eaten. I made the tuna salad with lots of chopped celery, some chopped up dill pickle, maybe some slivered almonds or walnut meats, and of course, a can of tuna packed in water, all finished off with a dollop of regular mayo. Delicious. And very low in carbohydrates. But too fatty. There's a better recipe for tuna salad in the back of this book.

Another lunch—my "very busy day" lunch—was a couple of slices of American or Swiss cheese, rolled up inside or around two or three slices of best-quality boiled ham, perhaps with a slather of mustard somewhere in the middle, eaten as a finger-food roll-up or with a knife and fork.

Eating something small with a knife and fork on a small plate stretches out the process, and fools the eye and the palate. For the same reason, place it on a small plate instead of a big one. I told myself that it was no different than a ham and cheese sandwich without the bread. And two or three slices of deli meat didn't seem to be overdoing it— some deli sandwiches contain six or eight slices of meat and nearly as many of cheese. I don't want to pan this one too much, because it actually is a tasty, low calorie bread-less "sandwich" for those days when there just isn't enough time for a sit down meal, or when you really want to cut your intake to the bone for a day or two. Just don't make it a habit! Unfortunately for me, knowing that it contains zero carbs, I also ate it as a snack, and the fat got me!

Dinner was fish or chicken, broccoli, Swiss chard or collard greens, maybe a tablespoon of baked squash for a treat, and tea. I drank lots of tea, morning noon and night.

Snacks were always either celery, peanuts, olives, or cheese , perhaps too, a chunk of mozzarella, Swiss, cheddar, or sharp cheese with jalapeno pepper bits in it. I was never hungry.

> *Fats provide nine calories per gram as compared to carbohydrates which furnish four calories per gram. Some authorities state that weight for weight, replacing dietary fat with complex carbohydrates means we are consuming fewer calories. True enough, but they overlook the reality of it. The dangers of a fatty diet aside, eating carbohydrates instead of fat raises blood sugar quicker and higher, triggering insulin production to lower it, which in turn induces hunger (Again, the old Chinese meal syndrome.) and increases blood fats. With all their dangers for modern man, where assuaging hunger is concerned, fats reign supreme. But please don't get the idea that I am advising you to select fats over starches. As you will see, there are other choices.*

My daily carbohydrate intake was not zero however. It doesn't have to be. You can lose weight pretty fast just limiting yourself to thirty or forty grams of carbohydrate a day. (I'll tell you how farther on—and you won't have to resort to nearly all fats like I did.) In the months from June to November of that year, my carbohydrate intake probably never exceeded twenty to thirty grams per day. I dropped forty-five pounds of body weight in under six months.

With my breakfast omelet, I allowed myself one piece of Wasa bread or Rye Vita—crisp, whole grain wafers that contain variably seven to eleven grams of carbohydrate, depending on the type of flour they're made from—multi-grain; eleven grams, light rye; seven grams. Guess which I chose. That was all the "bread" that I ate for the entire day.

I became so enthusiastic, that it rubbed off on some of my weight-conscious friends. Phil labeled my lunch-time tuna salad "Tom's Tuna Tsalad", and added it to his own lunch list. Peter modified my egg white and tomato omelet to include a slice of no-fat American cheese instead of the cream cheese that I dolloped on before folding it in half and plating it. Not as tasty, but virtually fat-free.

The pounds fell away. If you recall, I said I weighed upwards of 200 pounds at the start. That was in June. By the time I officially retired from medical practice in November, I weighed in at 155, and was flirting with 150, exactly what I had weighed in medical school. I had shed about 23 percent of my total body weight. And although I looked like death warmed-over because of losing that much weight in so short a span of time, I was feeling great.

There was a symbolic victory, too. As I got skinnier I began to feel energetic, running for buses with ease and taking stairs two at a time. My body was more flexible. My thighs were thin. When I crossed my legs, my top thigh flopped over the other one with room to spare. Tying my shoes was a snap. I could even do it without sitting down. The bucket seat in my car now offered more than enough room, even when I was wearing a topcoat. I walked the streets faster. I shunned escalators and took stairs. My knees stopped hurting. All those postural muscles previously occupied with just keeping me upright and getting me and my blubber through the day were now freed up for other activities.

I felt like I was returning to the ways (dare I say "days"?) of my youth. I started to look at motorcycles on the web (I rode one in my salad days). My prediction was coming true. I *wanted* to exercise, *wanted* to swim, wanted to jog a little, or to walk two or three miles.

Wanting is not doing however, and the road to Hell is paved with good intentions. I wasn't admitting it to myself, but emotionally I wasn't ready for a full commitment to an exercise program yet. I still had a distance to go before that happened.

When I went for my six-month check up in December, everything was normal except the cholesterol. The overall number seemed fine, but the HDL was a little low and the LDL was a little high.

"Nothing to worry about though," I was told. Total cholesterol was around 160. Allen suggested that exercise would likely bring up the HDL. (There's that "E" word again.)

"Keep it simple," I told myself. "Don't worry about total cholesterol too much. Aim for a test result where the HDL number is significantly higher than it was, and the LDL number is lower."

But how does one do that? The answer is simple, and I knew it. I hinted at it above. By exercising.

My doctor knew it, I knew it, and if you didn't know it before, you know it now too. But did I start? Not just yet. You know why. I didn't accept it emotionally, down deep where I live. I intellectualized it. I rationalized it. I fulfilled the definition of "rationalize" perfectly—I made comforting, untruthful excuses to myself.

I had obtained a finger-stick glucose tester, and was testing my blood glucose two hours after eating. I tested at least daily, occasionally two times a day, if social obligations or undeniable cravings overcame my common sense. With my fierce determination to do the right thing, overdoing it meant a few lima beans at dinner, or perhaps two Wasa crackers in one day instead of only one. With the finger-stick instrument, my glucose never exceeded 120, and the hemoglobin A1C proved it. It came back from the lab at 4.4 percent, well below our lab's normal upper limit of 6.5 percent.

But I looked like a cadaver. When I left the room, friends whispered, "What's wrong with Tom? He looks terrible. I hope it's not . . ."

When you lose weight rapidly you do look terrible for a while, until your integument (skin) rearranges itself and shrinks a bit to fit the new you. Exercise will help fill out the baggy sack you're now living in, along with helping to return the HDL/LDL cholesterol to a more healthful ratio.

But I was hitting myself with a double whammy. In addition to not exercising, I was consuming a diet high in fats. Meals and snacks alike were fatty. I don't mean bacon, pork chops, gravies and marbled steaks, although I ate those occasionally as well. It was the sneaky every day fat—cheeses, eggs, butter.

So, because I wasn't exercising, attaining that more healthful ratio of high HDL/low LDL cholesterol was going to come later rather than sooner. I told myself, "Those numbers will change as soon as . . ."

But there was always something to distract me—to deter me from the straight and narrow. After I said goodbye to my patients, I was too busy winding down. I felt so good to be down to fighting trim that I again put off exercising. I was thriving—on a diet only a timber wolf should eat.

A few weeks after I said goodbye to my last patient I started on something I had been wanting to do for years. I began to write fiction, and became so obsessed that I sat at my desk six to eight hours a day. I never gave a thought to the fact that I went from being an office potato to being a computer potato. I had discovered the computer magic of instant editing. Short stories poured out of me. Another fascinating distraction to keep me away from the gym.

Chapter summary: things to think about

My own weight loss diet; how I did it.

Complex carbohydrates, while better than sweet
    sugars because they are digested more slowly, they
    are still sugars and are digested into the bloodstream
    as such.

Both complex carbohydrates and sweet sugars are
    changed into glucose in order to be transported
    across the intestinal wall into the bloodstream.

Do not use the Food Pyramid as a guide to healthy
    eating.

Fats provide nine calories per gram as compared to
    carbohydrates, which furnish four calories per gram.

Continuation of my weight-loss history with lessons I
    learned.

The "new me".

Rationalizing the truth away.

Be careful what you wish for.

7

Blood Sugar, diet supplements, Glycemic Index

Somewhere along the way, I made two important dietary discoveries. I want to tell you about both, because they are vitally important to all diabetics and overweight people. The first is a nutrition database called the glycemic index, the other is a food supplement capsule, hydroxy-citric acid with chromium.

"But you're a doctor," you might say. "Didn't you already know about them?"

You might well ask. When I went to medical school— not all that long ago by the way, "Nutrition" was a once-weekly elective class of two hours. I remember the nutritionist who gave the lectures telling us that cucumber had no significant food value, and was therefore not fit for human consumption. Ditto pickles. Fiber was something you made into twine and rope. What they stressed, and what we took out of that "nutrition" course was, "Tell your patients to eat a balanced diet". Good advice, but it's taken us forty-plus years to begin to start to understand what a balanced diet is. And as a nation, we're not there yet.

The Glycemic Index, what is it?

The glycemic index is a database that lists which foods

raise blood sugar faster and higher (or slower and lower) than an arbitrary reference food, which is usually bread. Because it is such a universal food, and because its sugars and starches are so readily available to the bloodstream, bread is given a value of 100. Not that bread raises blood sugar by 100 points. Using a value of 100 for bread is just a way of establishing a benchmark number to compare one food to another. The reason bread was chosen as the benchmark is because it is such a universal food and because compared to other non-sweet starches, it is so efficient at raising blood glucose. Bread is also a perfect choice because other foods can be either below bread or above it on the glycemic index scale, giving us a more useful tool because it can cover a wider spectrum of foods. By choosing foods with low glycemic indices, we have a broader, safer variety of dietary choices.

Some glycemic value lists use glucose itself as a benchmark, and give it an arbitrary value of 50. But because bread is a real, everyday food, I believe that using bread at a value of 100 is more useful, and this is confirmed by its popularity as the reference food.

Here's why and how the glycemic index can help you control your weight and your blood sugar. The theory is based on the ease or difficulty of digestion of various foodstuffs. Some foods have a low glycemic index quite out of proportion to their actual starch content. Peanuts, for example, have a surprisingly low glycemic index of 14 or 16, (depending which list you consult). Roasted peanuts (the kind you shell yourself) are somewhat difficult to digest. Assimilation is slower and not complete. It is easy to see why they do not raise blood sugar as much as bread.

And consider the easy digestibility of peanut butter compared to that of roasted peanuts. This characteristic explains why the glycemic index of peanut butter is higher than that of roasted peanuts. I emphasize that we are talking here about roasted peanuts in the shell, not processed peanuts, for which all bets are off. In fact, all processed nuts, including "dry roasted" nuts, should not be eaten by anyone with glucose intolerance or heart trouble, period. While the glycemic index of the nut itself might the same as that for peanuts in the shell, industrial processing loads them up with so much hydrogenated fat and trans-fatty acids that they are almost a heart attack in a jar. And as far as *any* of the popular snack-chips are concerned, do yourself and your loved ones a favor, and vow never to buy another bag. (Notice the emphasis on any?)

How to Think About the Glycemic Index

In the Appendix, there is a list of the glycemic index of some common foods. I tried to create the selection based on foods we use in our everyday diets. It is in no way a complete enumeration. To date, a glycemic index value has been determined for well over three hundred foods. When you look at the numbers try to remember that they are not absolute values. Their purpose is to allow you to compare foods one against another, so that you can make an informed choice.

"Am I better off eating an apple or half a grapefruit?" or, "Since I splurged and ate that apple, to keep my sugar stable, which is a better breakfast choice—egg whites or shredded wheat?" (Even without the index, the answer in this case is plain, right?)

Some numbers appear inexplicable until you think about how they are derived. They are decided on by answering the question, "Compared to bread, how high and how fast does this particular food raise blood sugar?" That's what it's about. Let the numbers help you. Accept the values as empirical data and proceed from there. They are based on good evidence. This is not to say that you might not come across other lists that award different values for the same foods. So what? It doesn't have to be rocket science to be of use in our food selections. And you don't even have to know what a database is.

You may find that some values seem incorrect or inconsistent; whole milk 42, skim milk 46. How can this be?

We all know that skim milk is better for us, especially when we are watching our cholesterol. True enough, but the *fat* in whole milk provides less of a boost of plasma glucose than do the extra carbohydrates of skim milk. I do not recommend however, that you start drinking whole milk in place of skim milk. Isn't it more sensible to avoid the cholesterol-raising fat of 4 percent whole milk by sticking with skim milk, but just cutting down on the amount you consume? Contrary to the dairy industry's propaganda, cow's milk is not "nature's perfect food"—far from it, in fact.

This, incidentally, is another reason that even a quick look at the glycemic index is useful. It not only motivates you think about what goes into your stomach, but in what quantities. Which, along with an exercise program is the name of the game in controlling blood sugar. And in keeping weight off. And getting the benefits of a heart-healthy diet. This is my mantra. You haven't heard the end of it.

What is Glycemic load?

Glycemic load is a way to measure the *actual sugar load* of a measured portion of food. It takes into account not only the glycemic index of a food, but also attempts to *quantify* the actual increase in blood sugar levels that a particular serving provides. It's based on the fact that although a particular food might have a high glycemic index, its effect on blood sugar might be less than foods with lower indices because of its structure and density. For example, a serving of watermelon, a spongy watery fruit, does not provide the sugar load of a *similar weight* of say, hard candy.

While it's helpful to understand the concept, I don't believe that you should give glycemic load much thought beyond a common-sense recognition that the differences in glycemic load between foods is based on their density—how compact or dense they are. The reason you shouldn't try to work with it is that the glycemic load of a food is calculated as the glycemic index divided by 100 multiplied by its available carbohydrate content (i.e. carbohydrates minus fiber) in grams. Do you want to try to work with this in your daily life? My advice is to forget it. Just know it exists, and recognize that high G.I. numbers aren't the only thing to consider, and that in certain foods a high glycemic index isn't all bad. It's what happens in your intestinal tract and your bloodstream that matters. The danger of course, is when we tell ourselves, "Oh, the glycemic index is high all right, but the glycemic load is low so I'll go for it." Never mind that nice little rationalization! There lies another little dietary train wreck.

Hydroxycitric Acid with Chromium

"Wow!" you're saying to yourself. "Will I ever remember that name?" Sure you will, when I remind you that it's made from the rinds of citrus fruits. Citrus; citric. The "hydroxy" just means that it's not just plain citric acid but has been chemically modified a bit. It's combined with chromium, because blood chromium has been demonstrated to be low in diabetics, and is a nutrient essential to lipid and carbohydrate metabolism. I'll tell you more about it below, but first I want to say a word here about blood sugar levels.

The latest U.S. Government figures reduce the safe upper limit of blood sugar to 110 milligrams of sugar per deciliter of plasma, from the previous level of 115. Unless you are a doctor and can correlate it with other clinical information, knowing your fasting blood sugar (FBS) in early type II diabetes does not provide much (any) useful information, because even though your fasting blood sugar (FBS) is normal, the post-prandial blood sugar can spike to really high levels in early diabetics. In fact, this may be the reason that you were diagnosed in the first place, perhaps on an annual physical like the one I had.

We're beginning to understand that even a few hours of elevated blood sugar repeated daily, begins the insidious destruction of small blood vessels in the heart, kidney, peripheral nerves, and retina. It doesn't take much—a few hours every day, day after day, week after sneaky week, month upon month. This is one of the reasons I stress that blood sugar levels should be tested two hours after eating and not just before breakfast or before retiring.

Type II diabetes is all about the body's inability to process digested sugar. If there's *no* extra sugar in the bloodstream because we haven't eaten any, the blood glucose can look comfortingly normal, as is often the case in early diabetes. So if your doctor tells you to check your sugar just before bedtime, or when you awaken in the morning, it might be a good idea to get another opinion— unless (and this is important), the doctor asks you to keep a written record of your fasting glucose levels and report them to him or her. The reason is, that while fasting sugar levels are of little to no use for us patients, doctors can learn a lot from a series of fasting blood sugar levels when the information is correlated with the rest of the lab work.

The Two Commonest Types of Diabetes

If you are diabetic, remember this. With understanding comes better health and a longer life. So before I tell you more about this magic stuff called hydroxy-citric acid, and explain how it works, and on the assumption that many diabetics do not understand the underlying mechanisms of their disease, I want to offer an explanation of the metabolic failure in adult-onset diabetes, so that you will have a clear understanding of how to help yourself on many levels beyond just mindlessly popping pills from your doctor and fretting over whether you can eat a slice of bread as a substitute for some other indulgence. In short, a better, more useful way to think about your dietary and physical activity options.

I promised I wouldn't bore you with arcane biochemical details. We can leave those things to the researchers and the doctors who need to know them to provide good care. Let's keep it simple, and take it from the bottom up. Because many people do not understand the difference between the two commonest types of diabetes, I'll briefly summarize their characteristics and physical and metabolic defects.

Juvenile Diabetes

The main problem in what is called juvenile diabetes, ("juvenile" because it makes its appearance in childhood and puberty) is that because of an immune-system defect, the beta cells in the pancreas are destroyed early in life, and stop producing insulin. Since the beta cells are responsible for providing the insulin we need to process ingested sugar, the treatment for juvenile diabetes is always and forever, injections of insulin. Why can't insulin be taken by mouth? Insulin is a protein, and in the digestive process, proteins get broken down into the amino acids that comprise them. They are therefore not absorbed into the blood stream in their original form. So in order for insulin to remain insulin and be effective as such, it must be injected into the body directly, in order to bypass the digestive process.

Type II diabetes

I wonder if you think the next thing I am going to say is, "While *juvenile* diabetics suffer the loss of insulin-producing cells early in life, *type II* diabetics don't stop producing insulin until their adult years, and that's the difference between them."

Well I'm not going to say that, because that's not the difference between them.

In fact, most type II diabetics have plenty of insulin. At least in the early years, until their Beta cells become burned out by over-stressing them with ingested sugars, the disease itself, and the family of diabetes drugs that stimulate greater insulin production. Lack of insulin is not the primary defect in type II diabetes. The type II's metabolic defect is *insulin resistance.* Here's the explanation.

On/in our muscle cells, there are microscopic

"doorways", called *glucose receptors.* They facilitate sugar transport into the muscle cells where it's needed to provide fuel for muscular activity. For reasons we are only beginning to understand, in type II diabetes the glucose receptors throughout the body become partially or completely inactive, and no longer allow insulin to move the circulating glucose into the muscles (you might say insulin's main job'). Heredity certainly plays a role, as do obesity, and lack of exercise. As a result, the rebuffed sugar and its metabolites remain in the blood stream in one form or another, raising their particular brand of hell throughout the rest of the body.

All this is just a way for you to have a mental image of the defect in adult-onset diabetes, so that you will be able to direct your efforts effectively. Simply put, our glucose receptors fail. Glucose that was destined for muscle and nerve tissue to be burned as energy stays in the blood stream instead. Why does it happen? As I said, we don't fully understand why the glucose receptors fail, but research seems to indicate that inheritance and abuse are important parts of the cause.

How do people abuse their glucose receptors? Take a look at a fat ten-year-old child stuffing his or her face with hot dogs, hamburgers, other junk foods and snack foods laden with sugar and salt, tropical oils, chemical additives, trans-fatty acids, dyes and the like. Add two or three (or four!) cans of soda every day, along with ice cream, candy, cake and cookies, and the additive chemicals that are in them, and multiply that by forty years and 200 million people, and you will begin to understand why there are now over twenty-six million Type II diabetics in this country. How could it be called anything but abuse? If you think I am exaggerating, look up McDonald's and Coca Cola's sales figures for yourself.

So the initial defect in Type II diabetes is glucose receptor failure, or insulin resistance, as it is commonly called. We eat sugars and starches that enter the bloodstream as glucose, which then rides along in the bloodstream to where it's needed in a muscle cell. It knocks on the glucose-receptor door to get in, but the door can't open.

Enter hydroxy-citric acid. That's the first part of the combination in the dietary supplement capsule I mentioned above. The other part is chromium picolinate. Chromium increases insulin sensitivity. It helps insulin transport sugar into cells. The small amounts found in a typical diet are inadequate in diabetics, who have sub-normal blood levels of chromium. Furthermore, even for healthy people, most ordinary diets contain less than 60% of the minimum suggested daily intake of 50 micrograms of chromium.

Alarmist print and television journalism to the contrary, extensive research has demonstrated that chromium chloride and/or chromium dietary supplements are not dangerous even in doses triple to quadruple that of the minimum daily requirement, and you should know that diabetics especially, benefit from supplementary chromium in amounts of 200 to 500 micrograms per day. The mechanism of action of chromium is that it makes the insulin more efficient so that less is needed, which reduces the amount of insulin that the pancreas has to produce. Chromium also increases glucose receptor sensitivity, both of which result in better glucose transportation into the muscles and nerves, and less sugar remaining in the blood stream.

Three benefits of hydroxycitric acid/chromium

When you take a hydroxy-citric acid/chromium capsule, several things happen. First, because circulating blood sugar is accepted into the muscle cells instead of being refused by the inactive glucose receptors, the two-hour post-prandial blood sugar does not rise to as high a level as it otherwise might. And it returns to normal levels sooner.

Secondly, because more of the glucose we consumed is

now where it was meant to go to in the first place—inside
the muscle and nerve cells—that much more of it is available
for energy.

Finally, and this may be the most important effect;
because there is less circulating glucose, there is that much
less sugar to be transformed into its storage forms;
glycogen, blood lipids, and ultimately body fat and arterial
plaque.

So in addition to lowering our blood sugar and total
cholesterol, we start to lose weight. All this from a relatively
inexpensive capsule available in health food stores without a
prescription. Originally marketed as a weight-loss aid, you
can buy the combination over the counter in health food
stores as an all-in-one capsule. The dose is usually two
capsules a half-hour before meals, taken with a large glass
of water, but later on I'll suggest what I think is a more
suitable schedule.

There are other ways to re-activate the glucose
receptors too, but none quite so easy. In his wonderful book
on juvenile diabetes (Dr. Bernstein's Diabetes Guide, Richard
K. Bernstein MD, Little Brown, 1997), the author suggests
that exercising the large muscles of the body to the point of
complete exhaustion helps restore glucose-receptor activity
levels to normal, and that an exercise program which
includes programmed weight-lifting can be designed to
accomplish it. Something for younger folks to think about.

Chapter Summary: things to think about

Glycemic Index; how it can help you lose weight and control blood sugar.

Glycemic load; what it is and how to think about it.

Hydroxy-citric acid and chromium

Fasting blood sugar finger-stick vs. two-hour postprandial sugar.

Why FBS is essentially worthless unless the doctor does it.

A way to think about the two commonest types of diabetes; juvenile diabetes, and type II diabetes.

Glucose receptors, their function.

What happens in type II diabetes.

How hydroxy-citric acid/chromium combination works.

Getting blood glucose into the muscle and nerve cells.

Danger! What happens to excess blood sugar that's not used for energy production?

Another way to re-activate glucose receptors.

8

I'm Out Of Luck, I Manufacture Cholesterol!

The second part if the title is true, the first part isn't. You're not unlucky, or cursed, because you manufacture cholesterol in your liver. We all do. But the liver can't make cholesterol out of nothing, or out of heredity. It needs to have the raw materials delivered to it. The raw material the liver utilizes to make blood lipids (cholesterol etc.) is left-over blood sugar; that is to say, the blood sugar that remains in circulation after muscles have taken up all that they can, and our immediate energy needs are met—under the circumstances of our particular state of health, of course.

That superfluous blood sugar that is floating around in the blood stream after the muscles have absorbed all they can stimulates extra insulin production by the pancreas—and since it is insulin's job to clear sugar from the bloodstream one way or another, the insulin now sends the leftover glucose to the liver, where it is turned into blood-fats. In addition to its main job of mediating sugar transportation into muscle and nerve cells where it's used for energy, it turns out that insulin also raises cholesterol. Common sense tells us that if we had eaten only enough food to supply the immediate energy needs of our bodies, we would not have as much "left-over" blood sugar, that the body has to now turn into blood fats.

Something to think about when you've just about made up your mind to have that second helping, or if you decide that exercise is just for jocks and athletes.

> *Did I make it really clear? Eating excessive amounts of sugars and carbohydrates raises cholesterol. If you have a cholesterol problem, it's every bit as important to modify the starchy half of your diet as it is the fatty part. And this is one of the reasons that more diabetics die of coronary artery disease than of the diabetes itself.*

Here's a little summary of the actual mechanism. In the presence of insulin, glucose that is not taken up by muscle and nerve cells to be burned for energy is sent to the liver and immediately turned into glycogen. Glycogen is a storage form of blood sugar, and it can be stored in the liver for up to about eight hours, after which it is further metabolized, and released back into the blood stream as triglycerides.

Triglycerides are the chemical form in which most fat exists in food, as well as in body tissues. In the blood stream, they make up the plasma lipids, which of course include cholesterol, so that's where a good part of our high cholesterol problem comes from. Now you know why you, me, and everybody else who overeats, "manufactures" cholesterol. As I mentioned just above, knowing this makes it easy to put two and two together to help us avoid it, and helps us to understand one of the big reasons why diabetics are more at risk for heart disease than the rest of the population.

Rationale for hydroxycitric acid and chromium

If you are considering adding hydroxy-citric acid and chromium to your regimen, here's something else to think about. I touched on it previously. There is evidence that overworked beta cells in the pancreas (beta cells produce insulin) can become exhausted, bringing about an actual reduction in insulin production. It is thought that this failure of the beta cells can come about from heavy doses of the earlier generation of diabetic drugs that stimulate insulin production, just as it can from too much sugar in the diet. This is one of the reasons that the earlier drugs which controlled type II diabetics by increasing insulin production have largely been replaced by glucose receptor stimulants, except in severe cases where both are needed. As well as increasing the sensitivity of the glucose receptors, hydroxy-citric acid and chromium can indirectly help relieve the stress on the beta cells of the pancreas.

"But," you might be wondering, "why should I bother with taking hydroxy-citric acid when my regular diabetes drugs are doing the job very nicely?"

Well, in addition to this important reason, another part of the answer is, why take a powerful pharmaceutical when you can take a simple food supplement that may allow you to lower your dose of diabetic medicine, especially since we diabetics as a group are already deficient in chromium. Although nothing we put into our system is without side effects, food supplements in general have a much lower incidence of side effects than pharmaceuticals do. And as I emphasized, the chromium is especially helpful for diabetics for the reasons mentioned.

Too, if you are trying to control your blood sugar with diet alone, the billions of glucose receptors throughout the body become more efficient on hydroxycitric acid/ chromium, so plasma glucose can be more stable and less spikey. And last but not least, if you are an early diabetic *on medication* and are monitoring your diet, and decide to get yourself on a regular exercise program, if you are still a mild diabetic, you may ultimately be able to replace your diabetes medicine with the hydroxycitric acid capsule. That's what happened to me. But because this compound, like many other food supplements, hasn't been extensively tested in clinical trials, there is a caveat.

If you *are* on diabetic medicine, talk to your doctor before you start taking hydroxy-citric acid. He will want to re-evaluate your meds. You may find that after some weeks of taking the capsules your plasma glucose will be lower not just after meals but all of the time. Your blood cholesterol levels should benefit as well.

How to take Hydroxycitric Acid

I began by taking two capsules (the recommended dosage) a half-hour before my two larger meals of the day every day. After a month or so, between my walking and the hydroxy-citric acid capsules, my blood sugar was lower at all times of measurement. If you plan to embark on a diet anything like the one recommended further on in this book, and your doctor is kept informed, I recommend starting with two capsules half an hour before each of your two larger daily meals. Take the capsules with a large glass of water, and continue for a week or two, recording your finger-stick blood sugar two hours after both meals. Then re-evaluate the dose of all your meds with your doctor.

If, despite the hydroxycitric acid your two-hour post-prandial sugar is still mysteriously elevated, take a closer look at your diet. Read nutritional-content labels on everything you put into your stomach. There may be some sugar or starch sneaking in without your knowledge. One diabetic lady learned that lettuce is a free food, so being hungry and wanting not to displease her doctor, she ate an entire head of iceberg lettuce! Prepared salad dressings and pasta sauces are commonly overlooked sources of sugar, as are many other commercially-prepared foods that are not noticeably sweet. Sugar seems to be the one ingredient they all have in common.

And be in close touch with your doctor during this trial. He or she will want to know what is happening. Even without a big change in your diet, when you take hydroxy-citric acid and chromium, your body weight may start to go down a little because more of your ingested sugars are cleared out of the blood to provide energy, and not transformed into body fat and blood cholesterol.

Hydroxy-citric acid and chromium are not meant to permanently supplant a good diet-and-exercise program. Nor are they supposed to substitute for dietary common sense. Even though the extra chromium coupled with hydroxycitric acid is a great help, regular progressive physical exercise and a proper diet should be your chief focus. That's the real secret to getting your body back on track. I'm hoping that as you embrace the principles, activities and dietary changes outlined in this book you will not need to take the supplement except as an occasional protective, pre-meal "booster", when for one reason or another you cannot avoid dietary indiscretion. I'm hesitant to suggest this, lest that old devil rationalization kicks in, and those rare indiscretions become common every day events, but I promised myself I would acquaint you with you all the tools. Having said that, I have been taking a brand of hydroxycitric acid and chromium called "Citrimax" every day for the last five years with really good results.

Statins, summarized

Statins, originally developed for people who either had, or were at high risk for coronary artery disease because of inadequately=managed blood cholesterol levels, are today more widely prescribed than any other prescription drug. Statins are prescribed for virtually all cardiac patients because they have been proven to bring about a 20 to 60 percent reduction in LDL cholesterol. They lower cholesterol by inhibiting an enzyme, HMG-CoA reductase, which controls the rate of cholesterol production in the body, and also by increasing the liver's ability to remove the LDL cholesterol already in the blood but not yet bound to the vessel walls as plaque.

Considering that so many diabetics die not from diabetes itself but from the associated heart disease, I believe that statins should be prescribed for every diagnosed type-II diabetic whose disease is severe enough to require medication, whether or not they have clinically-proven coronary artery disease. The latest guidelines recommend attaining LDL levels of 100 mg/dL for adults without cardiac disease, and LDL levels of or below 70 for heart patients. I recommend that diabetics aim for the lower number, whether or not they have coronary disease. It is not an impossible goal. And the benefits of achieving it go far beyond lessened risk of heart disease and stroke, because the diet and exercise levels needed to achieve an LDL of 70 will likely end forever the problem of obesity, and all the premature debilitation that it causes. That in fact, is a secondary goal of this book. It is one of the many collateral benefits that losing weight to control diabetes confers.

Over the years, statins have come in for criticism for side effects, and for causing allergic reactions. At the same time however, long term use of statins has been associated with lowered risk of colon cancer and Alzeimer's disease, and there is also recent evidence that statins help fight osteoporosis by improving bone density in older patients. Considering the millions upon millions of daily doses taken worldwide, the actual incidence of side effects is very low. It is my feeling that their benefits greatly outweigh the risks, especially in diabetics.

Treatment with statins can reduce blood levels of the cellular enzyme CoQ-10 by inhibiting its synthesis in the body. There is reason to believe that adding oral CoQ-10 to statin therapy enhances the benefits, and reduces the possible side effects of statins. Impressions are that CoQ-10 may also help to maintain muscle strength. Discovered in 1957, CoQ-10 is an anti-oxidant enzyme made naturally by the human body and is also found in dietary meats and fish. It helps cells to produce energy and it acts as an antioxidant. Recent studies of its use in patients with congestive heart failure conclude that CoQ-10 significantly strengthens cardiac muscle.

It is undergoing trials in Parkinson's disease to reduce tremor. For tremors, it is given in large doses; 400 to 600 mg per day, as opposed to 50 mg per day as a dietary supplement for people on statins.

At the time of this writing there are five statin drugs on the market in the United States, with more on the way: lovastatin, simvastatin, pravastatin, fluvastatin, and atorvastatin. I'm sure that by the time this book goes to press there will be a couple more, which, in addition to being an illustration of the pharmaceutical industry's enterprise, is an indication of just how serious and widespread the problem of high cholesterol has become.

In addition to new statins, there is ongoing research which will produce more effective, lower cost alternatives. Even as I write, Merck has teamed up with Schering Plough to bring together in one capsule, Merck's simvastatin and a Schering-Plough drug that impedes gastrointestinal absorption of dietary fats. FDA approval is expected soon. The combination is said to be significantly more effective at lowering LDL cholesterol than any single product currently available.

Finally, there's a worrisome new report that in a large percentage of post-menopausal women, coronary arterial plaque does not appear as the characteristic localized excrescences inside arteries like those we see in men, but instead, develops as a smooth, invisible coating on the lining of the entire artery, *a coating indiscernible on angiography.* The first notice older women get of trouble may be the symptoms of a severe heart attack from complete and irreversible blockage. It is yet another reason to prescribe preventive statins in diabetics.

The 4-S Study and the Heart Protection Study

In the beginning of this book I promised that I would tell you about very hopeful evidence related to statins and diet modification. A notable long-term study, engaging over four thousand volunteers (actually 4,444 people) proved that a very low-fat diet coupled with a statin and an exercise program, not only reduced plaque in the coronary system of the subjects, but in the carotid system and in the brain. Amazingly, in a significant number of participants, coronary artery angiograms at the end of the study failed to reveal any evidence of the arteriosclerosis they had started with. Even more impressive is the fact that standard mental-ability tests administered at the beginning and again at the end of the study disclosed improved performances, suggesting that circulation to, and within the brain may have been improved as well. So much for the old idea that atherosclerosis can be halted but not reduced. There was a second large study which drew essentially the same conclusions (see below).

There have been several important randomized studies on the effect of statins on cardiovascular disease. Merck's simvastatin (Zocor) was involved in two: the Heart Protection Study (HPS), a large, multi-center study with a duration of 5 years conducted in 20,536 patients (10,269 on Zocor 40 mg and 10,267 on placebo), and the 4-S Study (details below).

The 4S study was the Scandinavion Simvastatin Survival Study. The effect of improving lipoprotein levels with simvastatin on mortality was assessed in 4,444 patients with coronary heart disease and total cholesterol levels of 212 to 309. The patients were followed for 5.4 years. The statin reduced the overall risk of mortality by 30 percent; of coronary heart disease mortality by 42 percent; and of having a hospital-verified non-fatal myocardial infarction by 37 percent. Furthermore, the statin significantly reduced the necessity for having to undergo myocardial revascularization procedures (coronary artery bypass grafting or a stent or balloon widening of a clogged artery) by 37 percent. One of the most interesting results of these studies was the finding of increased cerebral-vascular blood flow, (blood flow to the brain) which I mentioned above with the 4-S study.

Chapter summary: things to think about

How we manufacture cholesterol in our bodies

Dietary sugar and carbohydrates raise cholesterol too!

The effects of insulin

Re-activation of glucose receptors with hydroxycitric acid

How much to take

Ask your doctor first

Adjusting your diet: a first look

Statins

Regular benefits and side effects

Other benefits

Recent worrisome findings in post-menopausal women

Two important long-term statin studies

9

Ignore it and it Won't Go Away

By the time I started to even think about exercise, I was well into my retirement mode. I had plenty of other activities to keep me away from the gym; writing, playing my woodwinds, sailing, catching up on house and garden maintenance and traveling a bit. Unfortunately, none of the things I enjoyed doing qualified as cardio-vascular exercise. You may remember I said I walked a lot. That is probably the only lucky exception.

Because that's how I discovered that I had a blocked coronary artery. It started without fanfare. I didn't clutch my chest in agony like they do in the movies, or fall to the floor or pass out. It was just a little localized "unpleasantness", as the English say, in my left upper chest while walking along the street. When I stopped to wait for a red light, it went away. Not wanting to believe what my medical training had taught me, I managed to ignore it for several weeks.

That denial was the first stage, which is common to many coronary patients, whether they recognize it as such or not. The second stage for me was admitting it might well be a blocked artery, ". . . .but let's find out how stenosed (narrowed down) it really is".

Complete idiocy. It was that "Doctors are invincible" bug again. I walked even faster, for longer distances, carried packages, and searched out hilly Manhattan streets. To make a store exchange, I carried a ten-pound package down and across the east side of Manhattan from 88th Street to 58th Street, a good mile and a half. Yes, the discomfort was still there but it didn't get worse with that exertion, and it still went away at red lights. So I carried the ten-pound exchanged item all the way back again and walked even faster.

Fortunately, my wife and I were due for our annual physicals. I say fortunately because when Allen heard my story and examined me, he immediately made two phone calls. He called a cardiologist, and he called a taxi to take me to the cardiologist's office. Four hours and one thallium stress test later, the cardiologist sat me down in his office.

"I think Allen was prudent to send you straight over. The dye test revealed significant stenosis in one of your coronaries. When your pulse reached one-thirty on the treadmill your cardiogram went crazy. I want you to go over to the hospital for an angiogram".

> *Stenosis: narrowed but not blocked off completely (not obstructed, in other words). But— and this is a big but—a stenosed artery can become closed off at the drop of a hat—or maybe at the fast walking of two miles with a ten-pound package.*

I said, "Sure, Doctor. Let's see . . . .this is Wednesday." I pulled out my pocket calendar. "Shall we try for early next week?"

The doctor smiled.

"I've already called the cath-lab at the hospital. I want you to have the angiogram this week, Friday at the latest. If you need a by-pass, we can get you worked up over the weekend, so you can go up early Monday morning."

By-pass surgery? Now, that really got my attention. Noticing my expression he added,

"There's a good chance that you may get away with a

couple of stents, so don't start saying your prayers just yet."
     As it turned out, I was to come out of it with one stent.
It was barely two weeks after FDA approval of a new drug-
eluting stent whose effect has been to reduce post-operative
complications in coronary-artery stent recipients.

What is a stent?

     If you don't know what a stent looks like, picture the
little coil spring from a ballpoint pen. That's about the size
and shape of it, maybe a bit shorter and smaller in diameter,
although they are made in different lengths and diameters.
It is not a coiled wire like a pen spring is, but more of a
metal-meshwork tube that can be expanded in diameter,
inside the artery, to stay in place and provide a permanently
opened lumen *(lumen: the cavity in an artery, vein, or other
tubular organ).*
     To make the stainless-steel stent less prone to
rejection, the latest version is coated with a drug-
impregnated polymer. For some months after implantation,
the drug *sirolimus* slowly exudes out of the polymer coating
and helps the patient's body see the stent not as an invader
against which it must form scar tissue to protect itself much
like an oyster forms a pearl around the proverbial grain of
sand, but instead, as part of the body itself. It does this by
reducing the local immune response. It is an important
development, because with plain stainless steel stents, scar-
tissue build-up can block off the artery again. *It's called
restenosis. (Re: to happen again, and stenosis: to become
narrowed down.)*
     The drug-eluting stent is an important new
development because the chief cause of failure in stent
patients is just that—restenosis. After implantation of a
stent into a coronary artery the body's immune system is
alerted to the invasion, and scar tissue immediately starts to
cover and sequester the intruder. The FDA says that after
nine months, the rate of restenosis with the bare metal
stents was as high as 20 to 30 percent. That means out of

every one hundred patients who received an uncoated stent, nearly a third of them required further treatment because scar tissue had compromised the patency of the artery again, in some cases shutting it off completely.

But in a study of 1,058 patients after the coated stent was approved for use, only 4 percent of those who received the drug-eluting stent suffered restenosis.

In fact, that day when I went for my angiogram and was changing into my peek-a-boo hospital gown prior to the procedure, a diabetic man in the next cubicle reassured me that I had nothing to worry about; he was coming in for his sixth. Hopefully it was to be his last for a while, for he was eager to tell me that it was to be the new drug-eluting stent.

Questions remain

There have been some recent reports of "late" restenosis in patients with drug-eluting stents—late meaning beyond the period during which post-operative complications usually occur, which is to say three or four months. But even newer reviews reinforce the original low incidence of restenosis, so we'll have to wait and see. I'm encouraged by the more recent reports.

Chapter summary: things to think about

Ignoring chest pain on exertion - really dumb!
Stenosis explained
Stents described
Why stents fail
Drug-eluting stents and how they're designed to be
 less complication-prone
New Questions about drug-eluting stents
But even newer encouragement

10

How Angiography is Performed

As far as the patient is concerned, the angiogram procedure is simple, and essentially painless. The only discomfort is during the preparation of the site for insertion of the catheters, (usually the Femoral Artery where it crosses the groin), which is done under local injection anesthesia. Mild sedation is available for the asking via the intravenous drip in the patient's arm or hand.

I said that the procedure is comfortable for the patient, but it is far from easy for the surgeons. Under present requirements, before they are eligible to perform the operation, the men and women who perform angiography and stent-insertion have to train an additional three years after their already lengthy general internal medicine and cardiology residencies. (That means they don't start earning a living until they are in their late-thirties! Politicians take note!)

After the artery is exposed, it is prepared by inserting a small sheath to protect the entry site and help guide the catheters up and into the coronary arterial system. With the help of dye that can be seen on the fluoroscope, the doctor visualizes not only the catheter, but the exact location of the threatening stenosis. The narrowed area of the coronary artery is dilated by expanding a tiny balloon at that location, then the stent is inserted. Afterwards, the catheters are removed, and a pressure dressing is applied over the entry site. With the pressure dressing in place, the patient lies on his back for several hours before going home, for no stitches are inserted.

There is much more to the procedure, but it is not my intention to fully describe it, only to give you an idea of the mechanics—the nuts and bolts of it, so to speak, so you can think about it intelligently, and if it becomes necessary, to discuss the subject with your doctor with some basic knowledge under your belt.

Thinking about Exercise as it relates to coronary artery disease

When I went home the morning after my angioplasty I sat myself down and took stock. In a few weeks I was to start a regular exercise program that I will continue as long as I live. I was chagrined to realize that had I been exercising regularly to begin with, I very likely would never have needed the stent. The same might be true for you. There are no absolutes in the game of life and health, but it is just plain dumb not to turn the odds in our favor if it is within our power to do so. Contrary to uninformed popular opinion, we don't get sick or die by wearing out the machine. The thing that kills is *not* using our bodies; not sweating it out, *not* suffering achy muscles and joints from time to time, *not* getting out of breath from exertion.

The American military has a saying: "Use it or lose it." It couldn't be more germane. I don't care how old or debilitated you are, print it out on a card and stick it up on your bathroom mirror where you will see it every morning, because it applies to *you.*

Remember what I said about understanding something intellectually but not accepting it emotionally, down deep where we really live? That inability to accept the cold hard facts was the reason that the whole thing happened to me.

And if what happened to me has already happened to you, or if there is even a possibility of its developing by virtue of poor physical condition, couch potato-ing it, the presence of diabetes, or already diagnosed coronary artery disease, please give yourself and your loved ones the greatest gift of any that you could bestow—your own longer, healthier life.

Begin by taking serious, honest stock, by *really* seeing what you look like and in fact are—with all the varnish removed. And when you think you really and truly understand what is happening to your life because of inactivity, eating the wrong foods, and not being truthful with yourself, make a serious and solemn vow to do something about it. It is my sincere hope that a good part of that something—the part which supplies the life-saving determination, and the motivation you will need, will be found in these pages.

In my own case, among other come-uppances, I had to get it into my head to regard food not as a source of comfort, or part of social interaction, but as simple fuel—to weigh the benefit or harm of everything that I put into my mouth, and to try to see my body as a machine that to be at its best needs to be put to use, and provided with enough fuel to make it go but not more, and to be lubricated with sweat. Tedious? Not at all, when I consider what I got out of it.

In the eighteenth century, Samuel Johnson said the prospect of being hanged concentrates the mind wonderfully. Well, in my experience, so does the possibility of imminent, serious debilitation or death from cardiac disease.

To be honest, I didn't know how I would like exercising my heart muscle to some pre-calculated target pulse rate, keeping it there for thirty or forty minutes three or four times a week, going through the pre-exercise warm up, stretching out the muscles, doing the cool down. I admit that in the beginning it was difficult. I didn't like the beating of my pulse in my ears as I climbed the slope on the treadmill, or walked along the road at a rapid pace. Like most modern adults, I was better and more comfortable as an observer of physical activity than as a participant.

Replacing Bad Habits With Good Habits

But as I struggled along, fighting off impulses to throw in the towel and retreat to the sofa, something unexpected happened. As the weeks passed, I began to look forward to the workout. I was slowly beginning to understand the why of athletic endeavor, and the enthusiasm of regular participants. Little by little, my workout became a physical and emotional need. As with every good thing there's a corollary. If I skipped the workout for a few sessions I felt a little guilt.

What has happened, is that I have replaced certain bad habits with good ones. Psychology tells us that we rarely if ever break bad habits, and give them up entirely. It's simply too difficult. Knowingly or not, in the process of "breaking" harmful habits, we very often are not actually abandoning them and leaving an empty place, but instead are replacing them with others. It works just as well. Maybe better, because if the new habit is a constructive one, we've done ourselves some good. And the principle doesn't just apply to compulsive behavior habits but also to habits of omission as well, like exchanging a sedentary existence for a physically active life.

Second thoughts About Stents

In thinking about atherosclerosis, and how it manifests itself inside the arteries, I'm beginning to have second thoughts about the choice of inserting an intra-arterial stent as an initial therapy. *If a person has enough self-discipline*, it just may be better at the outset to solidly commit instead, to a rigid diet and exercise plan coupled with long-term statins. It is just possible that assiduously sticking with such a plan could obviate the necessity of having a stent altogether.

Since we are probably going to end up taking statins for the rest of our lives anyway, here's my reasoning. We know that if there is old sclerotic (hard) plaque in the wall of an artery, the artery also most certainly has fresh, soft plaque as well, as do all the other arteries in the system. This is borne out by large numbers of angiographic studies. Side by side in the same vessel, plaque old and new can be seen on the angiogram, the old plaque narrowing the lumen and compromising the blood flow, and the new plaque showing itself as almost translucent little bubble-like excrescences on the walls of the vessels intruding into the lumen of the artery.

And we know that even though the coronary arterial tree is studded with myriads of small new plaques, old, large plaques are usually the ones that receive the stent because they are the ones that restrict blood flow on stress tests and during exercise.

However, while old large plaques can significantly compromise blood flow, closing the artery down by as much as 90 percent, evidence suggests that this phenomenon is not what is responsible for most sudden cardiac 'events' (heart attacks), whether ischemic or infarctive. *(Ischemia; muscle-cell damage from lack of oxygen but not cell death. Infarction; cellular death.)*

Most heart attacks come about because the "roof" or "cap" of a plaque ruptures and then bleeds into the lumen of the artery. The sudden clot that forms inside the artery occludes the vessel and starves the heart muscle of oxygen-bearing blood, so the affected muscle fibers suffer oxygen deprivation. If denied oxygen for a long enough period, the muscle fibers die, creating a myocardial infarction. It is still controversial, but most cardiologists believe that newer, fresh plaques are much more likely to burst than old ones.

When I began to ponder this whole idea, I realized that after a patient has a cardiac event small or large, he or she is often frightened enough to change dietary and exercise habits drastically. And with the additional help of the inevitable statin, we now know that it's possible to

significantly reduce arteriosclerosis. And as borne out by
study results in quite a few verified cases, plaque was
virtually eliminated throughout the entire arterial system.
To me, that means we can now hold realistic hopes of
achieving really good results without a stent. The major
studies cited in this book, the 4-s study, the Scandinavian
Survival Study and the Heart Protection Study, demonstrate
it convincingly.

Because newer, softer plaques respond more quickly to
lowered cholesterol and a better HDL/LDL ratio, and since
they are the ones most prone to "popping their cap", doesn't
it make sense for a person who has had a scare to consider
going at cholesterol-lowering full tilt from the outset,
instead of getting stented at the first appearance of
symptoms? I'm beginning to think that the end result might
be better than having the surgery. A stent only takes care of
a single locus of stenosis in a single artery in a system
riddled with plaque. A vigorous cholesterol-lowering
program has been already proven to greatly reduce and even
eliminate significant plaque throughout the entire vascular
system. So what's the downside of conservative treatment?

The answer to the question is *discipline*. Specifically, the
lack thereof. It's the rare person (and the rare cardiologist I
might add) who has the discipline to take up a rigorous diet
and exercise program without the wake-up call of chest pain
and the possibility of hospitalization and surgery. Nor do
most of us have the courage to choose the conservative
route after a stress test has revealed stenosis. After all, a
cardiac event, severe or not so severe, is the reason most of
us get into treatment in the first place. So back in the
eighteenth century, when Samuel Johnson talked about how
fear concentrates the mind he had it right, didn't he? I'm
suggesting that maybe our fear could be put to better use
than just shaking in our boots over impending doom.

Understanding it now, I think that if I had it to do again
I would try the conservative approach before agreeing to
angioplasty. With close and careful monitoring by a caring
doctor coupled with a good dose of self-discipline, there's

no reason it shouldn't offer just as successful an outcome. The reason I say that is because ever since my own event I have been able to keep my total cholesterol in the range of 90 to 110, with an HDL level of 45 to 55 percent of the total. As you might imagine, it didn't happen by itself. It is the result of a greatly modified diet and regular exercise, along with a small dose of a statin (10 mg of Lipitor), and of course the most effective motivator of all—fear of death.

Intra-arterial inflammation: C-Reactive Protein

A good number of researchers and practitioners now suspect that arterial wall inflammation, possibly due to low-grade infection of the intima (the lining of an artery or vein) is the factor that not only responsible for plaque-formation in the first place, but triggers the rupture of the cap and the clotting of the small hemorrhage that then blocks the artery. Evidence for the theory is supported by elevation of *C-reactive protein (CRP)*, a blood marker that increases during many systemic inflammations.

It's been suggested that testing CRP levels in the blood may be a useful tool in the assessment of the risk of heart attack. A high-sensitivity assay for CRP, the *hs-CRP*, is now widely available. C-reactive protein is not too specific, because, like the blood sedimentation rate, it is elevated in many types of inflammation, and in infections, but we know that in cardiac patients, the higher the hs-CRP levels, the greater the risk of developing a heart attack. *In fact, studies have found that the risk for heart attack in people in the upper third of hs-CRP levels is twice that of those whose hs-CRP is in the lower third.*

Where does the arterial inflammation come from? Infectious bacterial suspects include Chlamydia and Helicobacter pylori. Viral suspects include herpes simplex virus and the cytomegalo-virus. It is quite possible that antimicrobial or antiviral agents will soon join other therapies to help prevent heart attacks.

The inflammation/infection theory is not universally

accepted. Time will tell whether low-grade arterial inflammation will turn out to be a major cause of arteriosclerosis, or only one of several possible causes. We do know that exercising and lowering cholesterol reduces hs-CRP toward normal levels. (The secondary benefits of regular exercise never cease to amaze me!) The idea is being widely tested in clinical trials. Along with their salutary effect on blood cholesterol levels, statins too have been shown to reduce arterial-wall inflammation.

The notion that chronic low-grade infection can lead to diseases not previously acknowledged as being caused by infectious agents is not foreign to most doctors. You may remember the heliobacter pylori bacterium as having been discovered to be the cause of peptic ulcer disease in a significant number of cases—a condition thought for almost a century to be caused by excessive alcohol consumption and business and life stress. Helicobacter pylori is now known to be a major cause of this disease, and treatment of peptic ulcer now regularly includes antibiotic therapy.

It is interesting to speculate that because diabetics are more susceptible to infections and to heart trouble, we might therefore be more likely to have low-grade arterial-wall inflammation than the general population. If true, this condition may be one more factor in the increased incidence of coronary disease in diabetics.

The bottom line

Now you can begin to understand my enthusiasm for the program I am espousing in this book. If results like these are attainable for me and for the people in those medical studies, they are possible for you. I truly hope that you will embrace these changes in your own life. If I had a choice of any gift to give you, I would choose this over any other, for it provides the greatest benefaction of all—a benefit without which nothing else matters; not wealth, not celebrity, not beauty. It provides the prolongation of life itself.

Addendum; Absorbable Stents?

Since I started writing this book, things have changed. Recently, small numbers of patients with drug-eluting stents are beginning to suffer restenosis, very likely because the drug that seeps out of the polymeric coating on the stent doesn't continue to do so forever, making it possible that the body again begins to see the stent as an intruder. I wrote about this in a previous chapter. But like time, advances in Medicine march on too. A major American drug company is on the verge of marketing a bio-absorbable stent, made from material similar to the absorbable sutures that surgeons use inside the body (collagen). In its development, they are already into the phase of human clinical trials. Like the coated metal stent, the new absorbable stent is impregnated with a drug to retard the rejection phenomenon. Along with the coating, after a month's time the stent itself begins to slowly melt away, and by the end of the first year or so, it has been completely reabsorbed, leaving only the widened, healed artery where before there was stenosis.

Chapter Summary: things to think about

History of a cardiac "event"
Stents: what they look like
What stents do
Improvements in design? - drug-eluting stents
Clinical results
How cardiac angiography is performed
Thoughts on Exercise as it relates to coronary artery
  disease
Replacing bad habits with good habits
Second thoughts on stents
Choosing not to be stented; a possible alternative
Is it worth a try?
Anatomy of an event
Old plaque and new plaque
The role of intimal inflammation
The bacteria, the lab tests
Another statin benefit
A new absorbable stent

11

See if you recognize this

We diabetics are constantly told that we must 'watch' our diet, that we must try to break the sugar habit. Stop eating sweets, stop eating bread, stop eating potatoes, rice, pasta. We are told we should make food exchanges, substitute a slice of bread with some other no-no. And count those calories!

In fact, there are so many dietary taboos, that if a diabetic were to pay conscientious attention to them all, he or she would have no time for anything else. Including getting a life. Worse, there are times when it is very difficult to say no to proscribed foods—meetings, parties, family picnics, weddings, first dates. Upshot? We tend to regress to our comfort zone and damn the long-term cost.

Since it's plain that nobody can possibly follow all the rules all of the time, what happens when we suffer a lapse of will, and indulge one or another craving? Well, several things.

First, there is a little denial. For a diabetic, it goes something like this: "I know I shouldn't be eating this wedding cake, but it's Amy's wedding. How many times is my niece going to get married for heaven's sake? Besides, just this once won't hurt. And it tastes so good. Especially with this wonderful French champagne."

This is usually followed by guilt: "I know I shouldn't have eaten that cake. And two slices! My sugar must be going through the roof! What did I do?"

And finally, acceptance. "Well, what's done is done. Tomorrow is another day. I just won't eat any starches at all tomorrow. I'll make up for it."

But do we?

The next time you go for a check up, the doctor admonishes you afresh. But if he censures too much, he'll lose a patient, or at the very least get a reputation as a scold. It's a fine line. So his lecture is gentle. He commiserates, he coaxes, cajoles, he understands. He adjusts your meds. He gives you a new diet sheet and an appointment in three months. You promise to follow it to the letter. You'll get yourself back to the lower dose.

You know what? It almost never works. This scenario is possibly the surest route to diabetic complications. How can someone—anybody—break the life-long habit of eating good-tasting food? (think sweets, fried foods and starches). And make no mistake. Along with the associated biological cravings, eating the wrong foods is also a habit. The reason is, that to a greater or lesser extent, we've all been doing it since we were children. Very early on, at our mother's breast in fact, food comes to assume the role of providing emotional comfort as well as nourishment.

So what's a diabetic to do with all the temptations, opportunities and occasions, tailor-made for gratifying the habit of reaching for the wrong food?

Once we have looked in the mirror and admitted the truth of what we're seeing, what is needed is a new way of thinking about the eating habit, a totally different approach to food.

I said somewhere above that habits are almost never broken.

"Oh really?" you say. "How about so-and-so? He used to drink, smoke, shoot up, snort, finish off a half-gallon of ice cream!"

Take your pick. Everybody knows somebody who seems to have kicked some vicious habit. Well, they didn't kick any habit. If they had, my statement that habits are seldom if ever broken would be hollow. It isn't. In a forest of psychological misperceptions it stands tall and true. With rare exceptions, what those friends who "broke" their habit likely did—and what you can do too, is something that works perhaps better than any other approach. Something that just might get you back on that lower dose of whatever. It doesn't take nearly as much will power as stopping what you're doing because you do not stop anything. Remember how your doctor explained how to do a bread exchange— substitute a slice of bread with some other food?

What I am going to suggest is that because relinquishing an ingrained habit can be as difficult as climbing Mt. Everest, don't even try to give it up. Instead, substitute a different, harmless habit for the bad one. Instead of leaving a nagging void, fill in the empty place with a good thing. If you're clever, you will work it out so the new habit is not just harmless, but is beneficial as well. The new healthy habit takes the place of the old bad one, and your subconscious will never even suspect.

How to Replace Bad Habits with Good Ones

There are three main aspects to making the switch. We are going to *change our activity level*, we will *alter our diet*, and finally we will *develop a new mental attitude,* toward food, toward physical activities, and habits.

In this chapter, we will concentrate on dietary alterations. Physical activities and their motivational stimuli will be considered in a later section.

Because humans aren't machines, there will be obstacles along the way, so to help get us through the dietary rough patches, the first thing we diabetics and weight tenders need is a substitute for bad eating habits and destructive food choices.

I've mentioned the concept of free foods. Low-calorie

fat-free snacks and menu-builders that won't elevate your
blood sugar, and that you can eat when the urge to eat
between meals is irresistible. We need to keep a supply of
these free foods at hand. If we're serious about regaining
our strength and health, they should completely replace, in
our larders, all the junk food that passes for nutriment but
that is instead, a cruel crutch that poisons us while it
enables the continuation of rationalizing our poor choices.

I don't have to tell you what the bad stuff is, any of us
who has ever tried to lose weight knows it only too well.
After all, it played a major role in getting us where we are.

My working principle here is that if we do not *buy* junk
foods, if we do not allow them into our homes in the first
place, the chances that we will eat them in a moment of
weakness is reduced dramatically. If we have to go out to
buy that jelly donut or that sugary latte' isn't it more likely
that we'll reach for something we already have in the fridge
or kitchen cabinet, especially if we have it in our minds to
change our lives? And if that "something" is a free food or a
low-carbohydrate snack?

> *A little side-benefit; when we make a healthful
> choice we rid ourselves of the sense of guilt that
> goes along with choosing an indulgence that we
> know is bad for us but that we eat anyway.
> Whether we are consciously aware of it or not, we
> are helping to eliminate the sense of surrender
> and hopelessness that is part of the whole
> indulgence cycle.*

Here below is a list of foods, along with some other
items that do not exactly fall under the rubric of free foods
but are so nourishing that we can use them as mealtime
replacements for potatoes, rice, pasta, and bread. They
probably should be called 'semi'-free foods. I do not suggest
of course that you attempt to keep all of them in your
larder. You will soon find which are especially appealing to
you. The supermarket aisles where these foods are located

are the ones you should be cruising, not the cereal aisles and the snack food, candy, soda and dessert aisles. Incidentally, the next time you go to the super-market notice that with some exceptions, most of the more nourishing foods are in the shelves along the outer walls, while the junk foods occupy the main aisles in the middle of the market. Why is that?

Some Free Foods

Fish, crustaceans, and shellfish of all kinds
Canned fishes like tuna (packed in water), salmon, mackerel, sardines and herring
Salad greens of all kinds; lettuce, escarole, spinach, red leaf lettuce, Boston lettuce, endive,
Celery stalks and hearts, plain or with a little peanut butter
(Note well! Do not buy the popular brands of peanut butter.They all contain sugar, added emulsifiers, and chemical preservatives. Buy only the natural peanuts-only brands. I buy Smucker's Natural, pour off the oil before using. The ingredients list says, "Contents; peanuts".
Fennel, sometimes called anise (celery family, large bulb at the bottom)
Cucumbers
Radishes
Cauliflower raw or cooked
Broccoli florets raw or cooked
Kale cooked
Turnip and mustard greens cooked
Swiss chard cooked
Mushrooms
Olives

Tomatoes in small amounts, (especially grape or cherry tomatoes, on the theory that it is easier to eat two or three grape tomatoes than to try to eat half of a regular-sized tomato and pass up the remainder.)

Green peppers

Cabbage, with vinegar and oil

Sour kraut, new and old

Most nuts (in the small amounts we eat them) but *not* salted, roasted nuts or sugar-coated nuts.

Coffee, espresso (espresso has about a third less caffeine than regular coffee). Learn to drink coffee without sweeteners. It will take about a month.

Teas of all varieties

Most condiments (with the following exceptions: ketchup, relishes, chutneys, *all* bottled salad dressings, and regular   mayonnaise)

The following are okay: mustard, hot sauce, Teriyaki and soy sauce, and low-fat mayo (for your tuna salad)

Dill or garlic pickles. Never buy home-style pickles, 'bread and butter pickles',or sweet pickles. They all contain sugar.

Bottled water, (a big slug of cold water can take the edge off hunger) The new Brita filter containers provide pure, good tasting water at a much lower price than commercially-bottled water.

Peanuts in the shell (6 to 8, no more)

No-sugar salsa—read the ingredients-label!

Tofu, extra-firm or firm, with salsa and a couple of nuts

Hard-boiled egg whites. Once a week eat a yolk.

WASA wafers or Rye Vita in small quantities
(one complete wafer over a day's time; 7 to 9
carbs.)
Commercially-prepared chicken, turkey, and
vegetable low or no-salt broths, or a bullion
cube iin a cup of hot water

I'm sure you can add some others of your own. Just
think of no-fat or low fat, low carbohydrate vegetable and
protein foods.

The idea of course, is to reach for one of the free foods
when the urge to snack is irresistible, or to prepare them as
part of a meal. My S.O. cuts up extra-firm tofu into little
dice-sized blocks, heats it in a non-stick pan and serves it
with homemade marinara sauce and Parmigiano cheese. It's
a really tasty substitute for pasta, with carbohydrates
dropping from forty grams per serving of pasta to an
amazing four grams for the tofu. And it won't raise your
blood sugar.

While some of these semi-free foods are a little fatty,
and even contain cholesterol (sardines for example), all
these fishes contain a high proportion of monounsaturated
fats and omega-3 fatty acids, both of which actually help
improve the HDL/LDL cholesterol ratio, a good thing to
remember when scanning the nutrient lists on canned
fishes, salad oils, and the like. And remember that you won't
be eating the starches and sugars that also raise your blood
cholesterol via the insulin mechanism described in chapter
eight.

You might be surprised to see tomatoes and cauliflower
on the list. They probably contain more sugar than most of
the other items, but the amount pales into insignificance
when compared to the sugary junk food you will replace
with them. And both are high in anti-oxidants, as are the
other cruciferous vegetables—cabbage, Brussels sprouts,
and broccoli.

Tomatoes contain an especially powerful anti-oxidant

called lycopene, which is being recommended today as an aid in the fight against prostate and breast cancer. But even if they are not protective specifically to these organs, increasing our anti-oxidant intake from any source has to be a good thing. In summary, compare more than just the caloric or carbohydrate content of what you're giving up and what you are eating in its place.

Lessons to be learned from the Smoking Habit

Smokers are told that it's the nicotine that has them by the throat (pun intended) and that they must teach their bodies to do with less by wearing skin patches containing ever-decreasing doses of nicotine, or smoking fewer cigarettes each day. There are even sub-lingual tablets available. There's a new "breakthrough" patch or sublingual tablet offered on the market every few months. But the American Cancer Society says that only three percent of smokers successfully quit. Why do the quitting aids work so infrequently?

A large part of the reason is because smoking a cigarette is not just about inhaling the smoke from smoldering tobacco leaves, it is an entire chain of actions that have become habitual from long use—abetted of course by cravings for the nicotine and tars in the tobacco. The total smoking habit is a complex series of many small events which comprise the whole of it; pulling out the pack, feeling the shape and heft of it in the hand, shaking out a cigarette, placing it between the lips, feeling it there, pulling out the lighter or matchbook, striking the match, taking the first draw. When it is placed between the lips there is even a faint, pleasant odor to an unlighted cigarette. I know from experience.

With the nicotine kicker added in, that's a chain forged of kryptonite. Successful quitters (I'm one, thank you very much) have learned, perhaps accidentally or by trial and error that they must substitute another, even stronger habit for their old, comfortable one. That is why some quitters gain weight. When they feel the urge to go through the little ritual they eat instead. Or they chew gum. Or if they're smart, they get really angry about how smoking is stealing their life away and they go out and take tango lessons or learn to play the piano.

I'm not going to ask you to do anything as arduous as quitting smoking. What I am going to suggest is not without difficulty and a bit of sacrifice, but the difference in your general well being, body strength, and life-span makes it worth the effort many times over. Make your beginning effort with free foods. Commit yourself to replacing the starches and sweets in your present diet with the free foods I talked about earlier. Each day, substitute one free food snack for a starchy food or sugary treat that you might ordinarily eat. When you get a yen, have a free food snack instead. Drink a full glass of water and leave the kitchen at once, immediately occupying yourself with something else.

There's a section in the next chapter on how trans fats, sugar and low-cal sweeteners actually condition our taste buds to want more. When you read it, remember that the absence of sugar conditions the taste buds too, but in a good way. So substituting free food snacks does more than just reduce calories fat and sugar in your diet.

Chapter summary: things to think about

Lapses in will-power—how and why they occur

An imaginary case history entry a lot like yours (and
  mine)

Can habits really be 'broken'? Do they have to be?

Replacing bad habits with good habits instead of
  trying to break them

How to approach replacing bad habits: a three-part
  program

A list of free, and semi-free foods and a way to make
  use of them

What we can learn from desperate smokers

Methods; a simple way to get started while you finish
  reading this book

12

A Cloaked and Treacherous Enemy

Training our taste buds

Perhaps a diabetic's worst dietary enemy is the taste of sugar and trans-fatty acids on the tongue and palate. The same goes for people who are fighting a losing battle trying to control their weight. We now know that *sugar* and *trans-fatty acids* actually alter our taste buds so that the tongue and palatal taste receptors become addicted to the taste of sugar and salty grease, and cause us to seek them out— think French fries, corn muffins, ice cream, cake and cake icing, candy bars, burgers and shakes, sodas, hot dogs, pizza, snack chips of all varieties, and yes, that wonderful fat-laden, sugar-laced latte that everyone is so ga-ga over today. Good coffee it ain't. There's astounding newer evidence that our taste buds also become addicted to *artificial* sweeteners, like saccharine, sucralose (Splenda) and aspartame (Equal) as well.

What does this mean? It means that you will crave it, want the experience again, and usually do what it takes to have it, including rationalizing your surrender. The smiling teenager on the TV commercial munches away at a bag of chips and says, "Bet you can't eat just one!" Absolutely true!

Now you understand why. You can bet that snack-food manufacturers do too. So does the fast-food industry.

> *Dietary sugars have one more harmful effect that nobody talks about. They make skin wrinkled, by a process called glycosylation. In the presence of free radicals, which are always present in our bodies because they are one of the products of metabolism, dietary sugar brings about cross-linking (irreversible chemical bonding) of skin-supporting collagen fibers. So instead of providing flexible support for the skin as it was designed to do, the collagen underneath the skin becomes stiff and unyielding, making the overlying integument wrinkled and prematurely old.*

If you believe me when I tell you that diets don't work, or better yet have experienced it for yourself, perhaps even more than once, then you must take to heart the following; *we must get cheeseburgers, shakes, and fries out of our lives by getting them out of our minds. It is our minds we must change!*

What doesn't work

On TV recently, I saw a young girl who was part of a group enrolled in a sponsored weight-loss diet plan. She was at the stage where she could think about going out to dinner as long as she was accompanied by a monitor. As the two ladies sat at a restaurant table, her companion asked her what she liked on the menu. Making a little joke, she laughed and said, "I think I'll have the cheeseburger and French fries with a shake!"

I felt sorry for her because I knew by her tone of voice and the look on her face, that no matter how much weight she lost on the program she would probably never succeed, for she was still in cheeseburger land. She was doing the sponsor's diet, but deep down where she lived, she was still thinking about, and still allowing herself to *want* cheeseburgers.

The sponsors of the study never told her the necessity of taking her inner self to a new place—a fresh new world where cheeseburgers are part of a far-away past life, and are not even allowed into the door of our consciousness, because they have been replaced with delicious salads and the reality of a new thin and fit person. They didn't tell her because they themselves probably didn't recognize that what has to be changed is not only what you put into your mouth, but how you must come to regard food in general and its role in your life. Ask yourself how soon after the study is completed will our young dieter find a reason to go to a restaurant and scarf down a cheeseburger, fries and a shake for real? Perhaps the first time she has a fight with her significant other or a reversal at work or school.

Something Else That Doesn't Work

This may be the most important part of this book. I see diet plans on television with photos of delicious-looking milkshakes, smoothies, and steaming macaroni-and-cheese dishes that the sponsors say have been modified so that they are acceptable on their weight-loss plan—perhaps if the dieter is taking their magic pill. I don't care if they modify these dishes to the point where they contain no calories at all, this strategy will never, ever work. It is like eating just one potato chip, or smoking a cigarette with reduced nicotine. As long as dieters are putting macaroni, or sweetened milk into their mouths, there will come a day—a celebration, or a party perhaps, or an emotionally-charged situation, when the reduced calorie version just won't cut it. And their sugar and trans-fat altered taste buds will be there to provide the irresistible stimulus to indulge. *It is our minds we must change, not the type of macaroni and cheese we eat.*

And Something That Does Work

While we are substituting good habits for bad, there's one more technique I want to share. Keep a pair of two-pound or three-pound dumbbells handy. When you get an irresistible urge to munch, drink a large glass of cold water, leave the kitchen, find the dumbbells and do five or ten (or fifteen) arm curls, or some other light lifting exercise. Incidentally, if you don't feel like buying dumbbells, depending on your age and conditioning large or regular sized canned foods work just as well.

If I've convinced you that bad habits should be regarded as nearly impossible to break but can be successfully replaced by other, less malevolent ones, you're half way there. The key is to choose good eating habits and healthful food selections over bad ones. Again—not how much but *what*—attention to quality, not quantity. Example; one slice of bread contains 20 to 22 grams of carbohydrate. Six egg whites contain essentially no carbohydrates. Not that I'm suggesting that you eat six egg whites, but it illustrates the concept of selecting quality over quantity.

Make a list if you have to, and stock up on those low-to-no calorie freebies. Leave the fatty junk foods on the grocer's shelves. *Do not bring them home!* What have you got to lose for Heaven's sake? The taste of fatty acids and sugar on the tongue? A belly full of starch and fats, another lost notch in your belt, another skirt you can't get into?

What about parties, picnics, dates, weddings, and meetings? Office sideboards with plates full of bagels, cream cheese, Danish, and a nearby coffee urn? Begin by refusing to go near it! Ask someone who's preparing a cup of coffee for themselves if they would mind fetching one for you as well. You'll feel good telling them, "I take it black, no sugar. Or, "No sugar please, just a little milk."

You don't have to partake, you know. And no one will know—or care, beyond perhaps envying your self-discipline. One of my friends is a recovering alcoholic. He's also a party animal. He knows only too well the old observation that for an alcoholic, one drink is too much and a thousand are not enough.

When they pour, he allows about an inch into the glass. He holds up the flute, makes the toast with the crowd, or the one. He smiles, says something witty, and while the rest upend their glasses, he just holds his glass without drinking its contents. Nobody's the wiser. You can do the same thing with wedding cake. If you can summon up the courage to leave the fork on the table, no one except the bus boy will notice that you didn't eat even one bite. My significant other slices through the cake with the fork and just leaves it on the plate. But be careful here! She's had a lot of practice. And she really cherishes her girlish figure.

It's difficult to resist the "just-this-one-little-forkful-won't-hurt" ploy to allow yourself to eat the piece of cake you've sliced off with your fork, so be *really* careful. Because one leads to another. Until you've gained some experience and strength at standing up for your principles, and some enviable pride in your self discipline (and in your new body), it might be wise to leave the fork on the table, and not even pick it up.

And remember this, too. The "just-have-one-little-piece" temptation doesn't always come from inside our heads. Our friends and relatives urge us as well, and this may be the most difficult to resist, because they are often relentless in their desire to see us fall. Don't ask me why. I don't know what motivation drives friends (and even family) to want to see you indulge. Maybe it provides an excuse for them to do the same. Resist with all your might. Make up a story if you have to, but the best story is usually the truth—tell them that if you eat it you'll become sick.

What have you got to lose?

Give my method a try. This is another situation where you have nothing to lose except abnormally high blood sugar, a big fat waistline, and those dreaded life-stealing complications of obesity and heart disease. Don't try to *break* the high-carbohydrate food habit. Substitute a better one. Use your imagination.

Other Ideas to Get Your Mind Away from Food

In addition to changing your menu, part of the substitution can be additional mild physical activity (additional to your walking), or learning to make your way in that long-deferred musical or artistic ambition, or perhaps in a craft. Your entire life will be the better for it.

Somewhere in the back of my mind I think about trying Rosie Greer's needlepoint (Remember him? He was the pro football player who accompanied Bobby Kennedy on his presidential campaign. He's still going strong, by the way.), or maybe learning how to knit, so I can make a big colorful throw for cuddling on the sofa with my S.O. on winter nights. I'm sure you can think of some not-too-complicated or strenuous physical activities yourself that will get your mind out of the kitchen.

Chapter summary: thinks to think about

Dangers of trans-fatty acids and sugars
How they make us crave more by conditioning our taste buds
A not-so-insignificant addiction
How sugar causes premature wrinkling of the skin
The story of a girl who will surely fail when she has an emotional crisis, and why she will.
Change your mind along with your diet.
Replacing that bad habit with a changed mind
If you don't take it home you can't eat it
Some things that work to help you beat the bad habits
Some tricks for parties.
What have you got to lose?
A couple of ideas to take your mind off food

13

The Physical Side—Exercising

Back at the beginning of this book I said that I consider exercise to be the single most important part of diabetes control. I want to talk about it now. We took a circuitous route to finally get here, but the things we discussed—the two most prevalent types of diabetes, how diabetes causes heart trouble and contributes to obesity, counting carbohydrates and calories, how sugar is metabolized, how insulin raises blood fats (including cholesterol), how certain vitamin supplements can help lower and stabilize blood sugar, other supplements that fight the side effects of statins, the value and application of free foods in our diets, changing our attitudes toward the role of food in our lives, how our taste buds become conditioned by sugar—all are very important to understand if we want to live healthier, longer lives.

Diet, or Exercise?

Can diet alone turn the tide? Can exercise? As recounted earlier in this book, my own experience proves how easy it is to be lulled into believing that modifying our diet might be enough to significantly lower body weight, reduce blood sugar and bring us back to good health, especially if we enjoy a little early success like I did with my timber-wolf diet. But it is a fool's game. Just accept the fact right up front that neither diet nor exercise, one alone without the other, will allow us to reach the goals of a stronger, leaner body and the better health that we are seeking. If you think that diet alone is enough, sooner or later you will discover as I did that losing weight doesn't automatically bestow fitness.

So the answer to each of the two questions posed above is a resounding "No!". Diet won't do it alone, and neither will exercise—at least not the type of exercise that those of us who have not spent a lifetime doing heavy manual labor or training with weights will be able to do.

Right from the start, make up your mind to engage in both a healthful diet *and* regular exercise. It may seem a bit unforgiving, but it is how the real world operates—the physical world of an active, sentient life, shared within species-specific limitations with every creature on the planet. The two parts, exercise and the right diet, are like weights on the ends of a balance beam; in order to obtain equilibrium, both are necessary.

Exercise changes our body's physiology, as well as our shape and body weight. Exercise not only strengthens muscle, it also strengthens bones and ligaments, and arouses dormant internal metabolic processes that turn food into energy more efficiently. When bones are stressed by activity, signals are sent to supply them with more bone-building raw materials, and over time they actually get stronger and denser. When ligaments are placed under controlled stress, their attachment to bones become firmer and the ligaments themselves become stronger.

There are several main categories of exercise we should examine. There are others—passive stretching, and yoga, for example—but the categories below are the ones you should know about for starters. (Notice I didn't say "do", I said "know about".)

Categories and activities:
1. high and low *impact* exercises
2. high-and-low *intensity* exercises
3. muscle-building with weights
4. aerobics

(Note the italicized words in the list. There is a distinction between high *impact* exercises and high *intensity* exercises that I'll explain below.)

To improve our understanding of how one or another of these four general types of exercise may fit into a regular exercise program, and which types of muscular activities are more suitable for our purposes, I will discuss them as they come to bear on the subject under discussion.

High Impact Exercise

I want first to discuss low-impact exercises and high-impact exercises. High impact activities are those which involve sudden stops and starts. The sudden accelerations or decelerations put significant stress on joints and muscle attachments. Because of the possibility of injury, high-impact exercises are more suitable for those of us already well along in fitness training.

Except for very old people, and certain of the disabled, most of us can engage to some degree in one or more of the low-impact exercises like walking, swimming, stair climbing, bicycle riding and rowing.

Even for young adults it is generally recommended that exercises like running, or playing tennis, football, baseball and basketball be engaged in only every other day. It is easy to understand why. The repeated pounding of bones, joints, muscles and tendons can cause injury in the form of microscopic tearing of muscle fibers, over-stretching of tendons and ligaments, and micro-avulsions (minute tearing away) of ligaments from their bony attachments. To give the body a chance to heal itself, and prevent the injuries from becoming progressive, a day or two of rest is needed in between exercise sessions.

So high impact activities are generally unsuitable as first efforts for older diabetics, and for those who are overweight, or have other medical conditions, disabilities, or injuries that could be aggravated by the accompanying stress. In fact, competitive sports activities more or less define the term, "high impact activity".

On the theory that when some readers will have reached the limits of an easy exercise routine as encouraged in this book, they may be enthusiastic enough to want to find more suitable reading material to advance their physical conditioning, I will be emphasizing only aerobic exercises. Aerobics are relatively safe for even the least fit among us.

But don't assume that because low-impact exercises are simple, and do not require vigorous, sweaty exertion and pain, that they won't be very helpful. You may have trouble believing this but it's true; of all non-professional physical activities, walking fast over a prescribed distance has been shown to be one of the *very* best ways to lose weight, perhaps even *the* best.

This means that there is hope for you, no matter what your physical condition, weight or age. Because whatever your present condition is, chances are that you can go out and walk, even if at first only a little. In fact, if this book has a message, it is this; that no one who can put one foot in front of the other is so far gone that they cannot improve, and very likely to a significant degree. There's really no excuse for not walking. You can start by doing laps around the dining room table if that's all you're capable of at the beginning. Holding on to the newel post you can step up and down on the first step of your stairway, alternating feet, first the right foot up a few times, then the left. You can circle your living room, or your driveway or your garage, or your city block.

Astounding Benefits of Regular Aerobic Exercise

Here are just a few benefits of regular aerobic exercise. For starters, regular, low-impact, aerobic exercise builds endurance by keeping the heart pumping at an elevated rate for an extended period, thereby strengthening cardiac muscle. As you know by now, it also boosts HDL cholesterol levels and reduces LDL cholesterol, and helps to lower resting blood pressure. Older folks who do regular aerobic exercise have a thirty to forty percent lower incidence of stroke, and they live longer.

Exercise strengthens the bones in the spine, pelvis and lower extremities and improves the synovial lubricants in joints. Best of all, and this is something I haven't yet emphasized, it greatly improves one's sense of well-being. It has been argued that aerobic exercise counters depression as effectively as prescription medicines do. This is especially helpful in older folks, who may no longer be in the mainstream of social or occupational activities and feel left out and lonely.

By engaging in simple aerobic exercise on a regular basis we set in motion metabolic pathways that utilize nutrients in ways that a sedentary life cannot. Our bodies revive long-quiescent pathways that burn away body fat, and give us more energy for the exercises. In the process, we also shut down damaging, retrogressive pathways—the ones that in the absence of exercise turn ingested nutrients into adipose and blood fats, and ultimately into atherosclerotic plaque in our arteries.

The Nuts And Bolts of it

So I will begin here to outline the details of simple exercises, and how to get yourself involved, whether you plan to attend a structured class (advisable), or wing it on your own (difficult, but do-able with the advice and help of your physician and a good book on aerobic exercises). Your doctor will be glad to go through the book with you to help you select appropriate first efforts, and help you define your limits.

You might think that when you decide to begin an exercise program it is reasonable to believe that you are adding a new activity rather than replacing a bad habit. In the strictest sense that might be true, but in fact, you are substituting the good habit of physical activity for the bad one of sloth, (defined as "aversion to work or exertion; laziness; indolence"). Getting involved in physical activity on a regular basis requires a set of mental and physical preparations and follow-throughs. And just like the smoker's little ritual I described earlier, all those individual links of the work-out chain are habit-forming too, only this time the habit is in a good cause. Somewhere along the line, you will have replaced the unhealthful habit of indolence with the life-prolonging habit of exercise.

First, you have to set aside some time. You have to don your sweats, shorts and sneakers. You must warm up before you begin the exertion phase, and cool down afterwards, both of which should a include a light stretching routine after the muscles are warm. And if you arrange it so that your thirty or forty minutes of exercise a day can replace eating something, or drinking coffee, or couch-potato-ing it in front of the television, you are not only replacing a bad habit with a good one, you are getting the little free kicker of reducing your food intake in the bargain. And the new habit will be the stronger for it.

The operating principle here of course, is establishing a habit. Remember that I said that when I skip my workout I feel a twinge of guilt? That a need has developed? That's exactly what you should be hoping for. It takes some months, but it's worth the wait and the effort, because after that, you are on semi-automatic pilot. What a wonderful gift you will have given to yourself and those who love you!

If you are lucky (through persistence), there might even come a time when you might even look upon food not as a place to retreat to for emotional comfort, but as the fuel necessary to keep your system up and running, because that empty place in your life that you used to fill up with food will be occupied by an increasing sense of strength and well-being that you will not want to give up.

This is another of this book's underlying premises. It is

important to keep it in the back of your mind, for if you do, it will begin to influence your attitudes toward food. As your strength and stamina increase, you will begin to feel younger, brighter, and more confident about extending your body's limits. Even four to five weeks can make a noticeable difference.

Why We Want to Eat After We Exercise

There is a little exercise pitfall I must tell you about—a trap to avoid.

We are told that prehistoric man's dietary history was one of alternating feast and famine. After the antelope or boar was run down, killed and roasted, early man had a surfeit of food, and like carnivorous predatory animals, he and his family gorged themselves against the days when they would have no food at all. We speculate that this pattern—vigorous physical activity followed by feasting on the spoils of the hunt, became fixed in our genes and accompanied us down through the ages, and persists there today, long after its usefulness is gone. Do you see where I'm going here? This ancient conditioning is presumed to be one of the reasons we feel the urge to eat after exercising.

There is also a physiological basis for the phenomenon which will not be pursued here, but for whatever reasons, we do feel "hungry" after exercise. If exercise is to be beneficial in reducing that waistline, those thighs, and that blood sugar, we must find a way to avoid eating immediately after exercising. Although surprisingly not talked about very much, it is a common contributor to the failure of exercise to reduce body weight. It is all too easy to put back on what we have just taken off—and then some.

There is a little psychological game afoot here, too. We feel good about ourselves for having exercised, perhaps a little pious for having done the right thing, and we feel entitled to a little reward. Our clever minds can come up with any number of convincing reasons to treat ourselves to a post-exercise snack.

Do not fall for it!

The countermeasure is simple, but the practice of it is difficult. Drink a large glass of water and leave the kitchen at once. Take your shower, change your clothes, go out and mow the lawn, call Emily, play the guitar, finish that report. In short, remove yourself from temptation, *physically and mentally.* And remember this—with regard to temptation, to a certain extent, *out of sight* really *is* out of mind. If there is a delicious loaf of bread lying on the kitchen counter when we return from exercising, we are much more likely to succumb to its siren call than if the counter is empty.

"Just one little slice won't hurt. And what's a slice of bread without butter or jam?" Or a slice or two of lunch meat?

I have found that if tempting foods are out of sight in the fridge or cabinet, it is much easier to walk out of the kitchen without giving in to the temptation. And as we do it, we must turn our minds away from it as well, and toward those other activities.

There's an ancient axiom: "He who loves danger will perish in it." And an old religious admonishment that's more to the point. In fact, it's exactly on target. If you want to live an exemplary life, ". . . avoid sin *and the near-occasions of sin."* Remove yourself physically from the opportunity to eat after exercising, and in the process, (and every bit as important, if not more so), take your mind elsewhere too.

Chapter summary: things to think about

Diet and exercise must be a team. One without the
  other doesn't work
Types of muscular activity
A look at low-impact high-impact activities
Aerobic exercise
Walking compared to other activities
Ancillary benefits of aerobic exercises
The exercise habit: establishing the need
A little exercise pitfall and a work-around

14

Increasing Metabolism with Exercise

What exactly do people mean when they say that exercise raises, or increases metabolism? Underlying this simple phrase is a complete sub-specialty of science and medicine. It is a big field. Candidates for graduate degrees prepare dissertations on individual aspects of metabolism. Some physiologists spend their entire professional lives researching plant, animal or human metabolism. So while it is important for you to understand how and under what circumstances our metabolism is increased, and why it is desirable for our purposes to increase our metabolism with exercise, there's no way that I will be able to fully explain the underlying concepts in the context of this book.

But in fact, there is no need. Knowing that "basal metabolic rate" is defined as *"the rate at which the body uses energy while at rest, to maintain vital functions such as breathing and keeping warm"* is enough to provide a jumping-off point for those who want to learn more.

For our purposes here, there is no need to comprehend the underlying concepts, much beyond being aware of the wonderful fact that exercise not only raises the rate at which fat is burned for fuel *during* the activity, but that fat continues to be metabolized afterwards, when we've stopped exercising. Essentially, that's what is meant by the phrase, "raising metabolism". With repeated exercise sessions, the general level of the complex of energy-producing processes is elevated via the re-activation of quiescent metabolic pathways whose sole job it is to burn body fat. Normally quiescent in sedentary people, these pathways are set in motion by certain types of muscular activity, and the fat-burning continues *between exercise sessions,* as long as the exercise is repeated at frequent enough intervals.

Earlier I hinted that this important health benefit of regular exercise is seldom discussed on TV exercise and fitness shows, or in popular diet books, possibly because it is a bit complicated. But it is a really important ally, and understanding it will motivate us anew, so let's try to simplify it.

High-intensity/Low-intensity vs High-impact/Low-impact

In addition to the category of high and low impact exercises mentioned in Chapter 13, muscular exertion can be defined another way; there are *high-intensity activities* and *low-intensity activities.* Don't confuse high or low intensity exercises with high or low *impact* exercises. When you think of high-*impact* exercises, think collision, shock, percussion, as in tackling or being tackled in playing football, hitting a baseball, swinging a golf club, or snatch-lifting a barbell.

High Intensity Activities—Fast-twitch Muscle Fibers

High-intensity and low-intensity activities are defined instead, by the *type of muscle cells employed.* The two types of muscular activities may overlap. High intensity activities can also be high impact exercises. High intensity exercises like weight training, tackling the pass receiver or swinging a golf club enlist *fast-twitch muscle fibers.* These are different from the *slow-twitch muscle fibers* we use in walking, standing, and bicycling, in that fast-twitch fibers are physically shorter in length, and are capable of quick responses to immediate need, but become exhausted relatively quickly. They are the fibers used in swinging a bat or a golf club or lifting a barbell—activities that require only a brief, intense burst of muscular activity.

Low Intensity Activities—Slow-twitch Muscle Fibers

Low intensity activities, on the other hand, whether rhythmical or postural, like walking, stretching, swimming, and yoga, involve long, slow-twitch muscle fibers—fibers that are capable of a slow steady output over an extended period. The skeletal muscles of our bodies have both kinds of fibers. Is this more than you ever wanted to know about "muscular activity"? And why should it be of concern to you at all? The section following explains.

The Krebs Cycle

Here's why the distinction between high and low intensity muscular activity is important to you. Over time, depending on whether you engage in high-intensity activities or low-intensity activities, your internal chemistry begins to change the way it produces the energy necessary for the task. To provide energy for the type of muscle cells used in walking for example, the body switches over to a system of supplying energy called *lipolysis,* (lipo = fat, lysis = breaking down or disintegration of; often called 'burning fat'). Among physiologists this process is called by another name; the Krebs cycle. The Krebs cycle is an internal, enzyme-driven "energy engine" that turns body fats into energy. It was discovered by Hans Krebs, a German biochemist working in Great Britain, and is named for him.

A Crucial Difference

For reasons I won't go into here, *fast*-twitch fibers—the ones used in high-intensity muscular activities—prefer *carbohydrate* as the substrate (source material) for their energy needs. Low-intensity exercises utilize the longer "slow-twitch" muscle fibers that prefer *fat* as their source, and the Krebs cycle is activated to provide it.

So if we want to lose weight, it helps to know which types of activities activate this fat-burning energy pathway, so we don't waste time or energy engaged in activities that burn carbohydrates.

It turns out that walking fast is an ideal way to activate the Krebs cycle—one of the best, in fact.

In order for lipolysis to begin to burn off body fat, it takes about fifteen to twenty minutes of steady, low-intensity exercise. (Incidentally, whenever I mention low-intensity exercise or activity, think "fast walking".)

Because the Krebs cycle exclusively hunts out fat to use as its substrate (fuel), it begins with the most-quickly and easily available fats. These happen to be the blood fats, especially LDL cholesterol. They get burned off first, improving that all-important HDL/LDL ratio in the process. This is the reason for the little 15-minute delay in burning off our body fats—the Krebs cycle is burning away those blood fats first.

It isn't difficult to see that thirty or forty minutes of fast walking, biking, or swimming can be more efficacious for losing weight than certain more-vigorous types of activities that do not activate the Krebs cycle.

> *Here's a short summary of what we've learned about the Krebs Cycle and fat-burning.*
>
> *If you are walking fast on a treadmill, or a pavement or road, or riding your bike, after 15 to 20 minutes, the long, slow-twitch muscle fibers used in these activities will have burned up all the readily available fatty energy sources in the bloodstream and in the muscles, and the Krebs cycle will then turn to burning the body fat to supply the needed energy. If your workout lasts for one-half to one hour, you are metabolizing body fat.*
>
> *If the exercise that activated the Krebs cycle is discontinued for a period of days, the body slowly reverts to its old way of metabolizing excess dietary carbohydrates, by turning them into blood fats and then to adipose. Remember how insulin causes the liver to metabolize left-over blood glucose into blood fats and then to body fat? Well, that's what your metabolism reverts to.*

Here's an extra benefit of activating the Krebs cycle that I briefly mentioned above. Because the Krebs cycle's *first* choice for its fuel is blood fats, regular aerobic exercise changes the ratio of HDL cholesterol to LDL cholesterol—raising HDL and lowering LDL, *even in the absence of bodily weight loss.* And of course, if you are eating properly along with the exercising, body fat will begin to melt away.

We should all have our sweat shirts stenciled with, "Hooray for the Krebs Cycle!"

Chapter summary; Things to think about

Increasing metabolic rate with exercise
What is metabolic rate? And what does it mean to
 'increase your metabolism'?
High-intensity or low-intensity exercises; differences
Fast-twitch muscle fibers
Slow-twitch muscle fibers
Burning body fats: what does it?
The Krebs cycle; what it is, what it does
How to activate it
Lipolysis, "burning" fat
Low-intensity activities best for burning fats
Summary of the Krebs cycle
Lower bad cholesterol even before you start losing
 weight

15

The Truth Shall Set You Free

Facing Facts

Along with the attention to diet and exercise, there's another component of losing weight and avoiding the complications of diabetes that I haven't mentioned yet. It is something so important that without it, none of the aforementioned knowledge or techniques will help you very much, but with it, the battle is already half yours. It must be a part of any effort to regain health and fitness.

It is just this; making a real effort to see the truth about yourself, and not pleasing your emotional needs with comforting fictions. I must admit at the outset that it is difficult. It necessitates our willingness to coldly see and admit the real facts about our day-to-day activity level, our food intake and our body's actual physical shape, weight, and state of conditioning, and not comfort ourselves with dishonest platitudes.

We all rationalize. It's a human trait. And it's not a weakness, or a failing. It's just that in an effort to keep us comfortable, our natures often hide the awful truth from us, and in some circumstances, this can hurt us in the long run. Remember the definition of rationalization? *. . . to devise* *self-satisfying, but incorrect reasons for one's behavior.*

Recognizing and admitting the truth is not all or nothing, by the way. It doesn't have to be brutal. Look at it this way; there is not a person alive who doesn't pass off certain realities that are simply too painful to endure. If we didn't, we couldn't live with ourselves or even exist as communal beings.

But seeking emotional and physical comfort at the cost of *all* common sense shouldn't take over our lives to the point where it robs our health and fitness away, shortens our lives and burdens our senior years and those of our family with avoidable infirmities. Unfortunately, this is exactly what is happening all across America, and the rest of the civilized world, as well. That's why this part of the book is so very important.

Physicists tell us that entropy is time's arrow—that without some intellectual and physical resistance, a little suck-it-up determination, along with the rest of Creation we're all supposed to end up as primordial ooze, homogenized and without form, like stuff in the city dump. By all that we love and cherish in this world, we must not allow ourselves to go that route.

Remember when I described taking that long, naked look in my bedroom mirror? Well, you owe that little revelation to yourself, as well. It might be disquieting, but it's a beginning, isn't it? Think of it as the 'before', of your 'before and after'. And don't forget that once you commit yourself to start your journey, and actually do so, you will discover milestones of progress (increased self-esteem and those feelings of well-being and conditioning I mentioned) that will surprise and delight you as they reinforce the new habit.

Doing it yourself versus going to a trainer

For patients with diagnosed coronary artery disease, most hospitals now offer three-month cardiac rehabilitation programs that are covered by Medicare. If you have had a cardiac 'event', and are of Medicare age, that's the first place to look. Your internist or cardiologist will know.

If finances allow, there is one responsibility that you should hand off. With the exception of establishing a walking routine, which you can and should plan and establish yourself, and which I will describe in some detail, you should delegate the responsibility of designing and maintaining a progressive exercise program to a professional, if only until you get started. To begin with, just trying to understand and manage your particular limits is daunting, and can bring you to a full stop.

How fast do I advance? Am I pushing too hard, maybe endangering my heart? Not hard enough? What are the danger signs? How do I recognize them? How long should each session be? Should I exercise every day? What's the best way to warm up? To cool down?

And then there's maintaining the will to continue on days when you'd rather warm up to a nice cup of coffee and a bagel instead of a windy road, a treadmill, or a stationary bicycle. That trickle of sweat running down the middle of your back can't compete with comfort foods, and warm cozy places. It happens to all of us on occasion, even the most determined fitness die-hards. That's one of the reasons that going to a gym is a great help, especially in the beginning, until you have established a strong habit, and have a grip on your routine.

The fact that your trainer or instructor expects you to show up supplies the motivation you need on those days when you want nothing more than to stay in your nice, comfortable home. I promise that once you are warmed up, you will be glad that you decided to go. It never fails. No matter how reluctant I am to get up and out on my two-mile rapid walk or gym session, once I get going, I'm *never* sorry that I did. A conscientious trainer or instructor will not only set up an intelligent program which is tailored to your specific needs, but will help provide the motivation to help you carry on when your own temporarily deserts you. But even if I do it alone on a cold and windy road, and have to screw up my courage to go out, I'm always glad I made the decision to go.

So if at all possible, let the gym and trainer carry some of the weight. That's what they are paid to do. In a sense, all you have to do is show up. Just from day-to-day repetition of the routines you will begin to learn them all by heart, even if you don't become mentally involved and just go through the motions (with a will, of course). You will be taught how to safely push your limits during the exercises, and how to develop safe routines to warm up, stretch out, and cool down. A side-benefit here is that if you are able to get your doctor's recommendation to enter the three-month cardiac rehabilitation mentioned above, the sequence of warm-ups, exercises, and cool-downs will serve you very well in your own long-term agenda after the rehab program is completed.

As the exercise routine settles into your psyche, and you finish the two or three-month program and go on your way, you will have developed a semi-automatic workout habit that you will want to continue on your own. Bear in mind though, that unless you become really dedicated, it is probable that your new automatic pilot may require a bit of a tweak once in a while to get you back on track. That's why I called it a *semi-automatic* habit. Whenever you feel yourself slipping into the old easy ways again, fire up your determination by asking a trainer to guide you back onto the right path, or go back to the gym for some sessions with your old trainer. Many hospitals that offer three-month cardiac rehab programs also offer month-by-month extensions at low cost (the extended programs are not covered by Medicare but are well worth the small cost).

A Disclaimer – with a twist

If you are over the age of forty-five, or have heart trouble or hypertension, non-supervised exertion can be dangerous. I do not mean to suggest that you should give up the idea—just the opposite, in fact. I've gone to great lengths to convince you that in my opinion, aerobic exercise is far and away the single most important element of your diabetes care, and if you are a heart patient, of your cardiac care. More than anything else, it is the thing that will make the biggest difference in your life. Regular exercise will raise your HDL, lower your LDL, help stabilize your blood sugar, and if you are diligent, very possibly allow you to lower your daily dose of medications. Exercise will firm up your body, improve your posture, raise your energy level, help you to lose weight, get stronger, feel better, achieve better balance, help prevent bone loss if you're older, lubricate your joints, and on and on. If that isn't enough reason to get started, I don't know what is. But do the sensible thing and get clearance from your physician before you cast off.

Here's the little "twist". Within the bounds of common sense, there is one exercise for which you don't need to get medical approval, or make any special preparations to do. And it happens to be one of the very best things you can do for yourself.

Unless it makes you dizzy or weak even to pull yourself up out of a chair, you can walk all you want without fear of doing yourself harm, even if in the beginning you are just walking around the dining room table. Just be sure to set a comfortable pace, and don't get carried away with enthusiasm and overdo it, especially in the beginning. Be certain to let your doctor know you are walking. And be sure to tell the doctor if there is any chest discomfort or shortness of breath from the activity.

Chapter summary; things to think about

The importance of facing facts
Fact versus fiction
Acceptance versus rationalization; seeing yourself as
 you really are
Making the commitment; keeping the goals in sight
Advantages of going to a gym or having a trainer
Motivation and how to keep it
Learning the routines
Developing the habit: the semi-automatic pilot
You can do it yourself
A disclaimer with a twist

16

The Skinny on Walking

It doesn't matter what your age, weight, or physical condition are, I'm going to go on record, and say that rapid walking is the single best exercise you can do. It is under-rated as an exercise modality because it is so commonplace in our lives—it's what gets us from place to place in our everyday lives. But in addition to the fact that walking fast is the very best way to lose weight, there is no other activity that gives such great rewards for so little effort, is so available at any hour or location, and that needs no specialized equipment. And you don't need a doctor's permission to do it. In fact, telling your doctor that you are walking a mile or two every day will encourage him immeasurably. But it has to be fast. Brisk walking burns almost as many calories as jogging over the same distance and poses far less risk for injury to muscle, tendons and bone.

Let's be clear: jogging burns more calories per minute, but over an equal distance, brisk walking burns almost the same number of calories as jogging does because it takes longer to cover that distance.

Equipment - Clothing

For walking, layered clothing suitable to the season and outside temperature and a pair of supportive, comfortable shoes are all that you need. Walking will get you where you are going, and provide a healthful, safe and effective workout, without the necessity of a formal warm-up or cooling-down routine.

Our legs are the first part of us to fail as we grow older. To illustrate how true this is, ask any old person what their chief physical difficulty is? I can suggest almost without fear of contradiction, that their answer will be, "Walking—getting about, climbing stairs".

Walking not only builds muscle in our lower extremities, it strengthens shoulder, hip, knee, foot, and ankle cartilage, and stimulates secretion of lubricating fluids into the joints. It improves heart action and pulmonary function, tunes up glucose receptors in the big thigh and lower leg muscles, and not least, makes you feel good. And you don't have to crank up your enthusiasm to get started the way you do with more strenuous regimens. An over-enthusiastic exaggeration? Not in the least. Just wait and see. And you can forget about seasonal affective disorder (SAD), that awful wintertime emotional depression that affects stay-at-homes who don't get enough sunshine.

The secret; Regular, fast Walking

Back in the Seventies when the jogging craze was at its peak, someone published an entire book on walking. I bought it because when I skimmed though it in the book store, I laughed out loud. As though humankind hasn't been walking for untold thousands of years, it actually explained how to place one foot in front of the other, which way to point the toes, how to swing the arms (Try doing it the other way!), establish a rhythm, and so on. There were entire chapters on walking clothes, walking diets, and walking music.

Notwithstanding such superfluous dissection of something that we've all been doing since we learned to toddle at our mother's knee, I want to describe the kind of walking I have in mind.

It is *rapid* walking. If you take a look around, you will see that by and large, Americans have forgotten how to walk fast. Truth be told, except to get to the car, an alarming number of Americans have forgotten how to walk, period. For many of us, if we live in the country, the longest distance we walk is out to the mailbox and back, or if we are town dwellers, perhaps as far as to the curb to collect the newspaper, or sink into the car.

Big city people are fortunate in this regard. They have every reason and opportunity to walk fast. In New York, I can cover over two or three miles a day without even trying, always briskly, always purposefully. The rapid pace of New York pedestrians makes it easy. I can always find a reason to walk fast. And I often have to carry packages, groceries and the like—a collateral benefit that helps build stamina. The trick is to make up your mind to stay out of automobiles, cabs, and buses, and to take stairs instead of escalators for one or two flights. If there's no alternative to an escalator, I try to walk up the escalator steps as they travel along, (but that's probably just my over-enthusiasm).

In the country or the suburbs, try to park farther away from your destination at shopping malls and stores. Over time, little strategies can make a significant difference, not only in your physical condition but just as importantly in your overall attitude toward physical activity and in your feelings of well-being.

For obvious reasons, finding occasions to walk fast is more difficult in the country, so to get your miles in you may want to develop a little daily route. In my automobile, I measured off a two-mile circle, which starts from my home and ends up there. It ended up being 2.2 miles. You can do the same thing in the city of course. On days when I feel especially energetic I can lengthen the distance to suit by repeating a portion within the original route. When I do, I try to choose the hilly parts. Because walking uphill usually entails walking back down the hill, you should know that walking fast downhill uses its own set of muscles, which are a somewhat different group than the ones needed to carry you uphill, so although not as strenuous, it has its own benefits.

The secret to fast walking is to get outside yourself. Walk briskly. As exercise, strolling is a waste of time. Carry or wear a watch, so you can check your pulse. (For pulse measurement methods see the Appendix, but not now. There's also a section on how to determine your own maximum exercise heart rate, adjusted for your age.)

If you are worried that you might not be monitoring your pulse accurately, and are concerned about overdoing, here is a simple idea to help keep you within safe boundaries. As long as you can talk or sing a simple ditty (like "Row, row, row your boat" for example) while you are walking rapidly, current opinion is that your heart will not be not working too hard, and you will not be getting yourself into trouble. In other words, you are not out of breath. Be aware of the corollary; if you find that trying to walk and talk at the same time leaves you short of breath, it's time to slow down, or stop for a break and a re-evaluation of speeds and distances. Don't be discouraged by this though, walking increases cardiac strength and stamina rapidly.

You might consider this a good reason to have a walking buddy, but in general I discourage walking with another person, no matter how much you love them. (I guess that makes me a curmudgeon!) On my route I often see couples and friends walking together, talking all the way. What began as a fast exercise walk has turned into a stroll. The reason for the hike is forgotten, and socializing has assumed primary importance. When you walk alone you can set your pace according to your own abilities, and you do not have to consider someone else's limitations, superior abilities or interest level. You can concentrate on the level of your own conditioning, and day by day, you can push your limits a little, which is important to improving your fitness.

And walking alone provides the best opportunity to get in touch with your body, listen to its rhythms and to clear your mind of trivial matters, and yes, to enjoy the great outdoors.

By the way, if you have decided to keep tabs on your pulse rate, you will know you are improving your heart-muscle strength when after some weeks of steady exercise, your pulse rate after your walk be comes back to its normal resting rate sooner than it did when you first started your program. In the beginning, I kept a little diary in a nickel notebook of the ever-decreasing times for my pulse to slow to 80 beats per minute after I stopped exercising.

And as you become fitter, your resting pulse rate will be lower too—that's your pulse rate when you haven't engaged in any activity to increase it. The reason it becomes slower with increasing fitness, is because the heart's stroke-volume increases. As the heart muscle strengthens, each individual beat or stroke pumps a larger volume of oxygen-laden blood to the body, so that fewer beats are needed over a given length of time to push the same amount of blood to distant organs and muscles. I have a friend who is a bicycle racer. His resting pulse is an amazing forty-two beats per minute. His heart supplies all the blood his resting body needs each minute with just forty two strokes of his heart. Across the animal kingdom, species with slower heart rates are known to have longer life-spans. Hmmm.

To summarize; dress for the weather, wear gloves or mittens if it's cold (Mittens keep fingers warmer than gloves do. L.L. Bean has some really warm mittens in their catalog), and wear smooth, comfortable socks, and sturdy shoes.

If you can feel the toe seams in your socks when you walk, turning the socks inside out so that the lumpy toe seams are on the outside helps a little, but it's even better to choose carefully when you buy them. I've found that some brands of sports socks have nice smooth toe areas, with little or no bumpy stitching. This is especially important for diabetics, who are more susceptible to foot problems because of circulation deficits. Those seams can abrade and blister the toes. In warm weather, a peaked cap and sunglasses will help to keep the sun out of your eyes. In winter, carry or wear a warm cap that you can pull down over your ears. For the sake of increasing your safety on the roads and streets, choose clothing which is white or brightly colored, instead of dark or neutral colors which tend to blend in with the background.

If I have convinced you to use walking as one of your exercise modalities, make it count for something. Don't stroll along, hands in pockets. As I said above, that's not the kind of walking that will do you any good. Instead, insofar as you are able, really step out. Straighten up your shoulders and your back, thrust your chest forward a bit. It will help you feel the momentum. With the idea in mind that every little bit helps, swing your arms. Some walkers pump their arms with elbows bent. It's another good way to establish rhythm and pace. And keep your head tall.

If you're not used to walking fast, you might feel a little ungainly in the beginning, all elbows and knees so to speak. Maybe one calf hurts, or your ankle or knee is a little stiff. If you're walking fast and are really beginning to stretch it out, somewhere along the way you might want to stop and count your pulse, not as a worry factor but as a reference, because if you stop to measure it at the same spot once a week or so, as the weeks pass you will see positive evidence of your progress towards fitness because your pulse will be lower. At the top of the first hill is a good spot.

After a half mile or so, you will begin to realize that those minor aches and pains won't cripple you, and that you may actually be able to work them out along your route by stopping and stretching. By the time you have logged a quarter mile or so, one or two of them may have already disappeared. You might have the urge to stop and stretch your leg muscles a bit, because your body is beginning to speak to you and you are reading the signals. If it's the first time in a while, revel in it. It's exactly what our Creator intended. You're becoming a part of the great natural world. Think to yourself that whatever muscle soreness you're feeling now it will only get better with time.

Stretching

We've all seen runners leaning on a light pole or a tree with one foot behind, stretching out their Achilles' tendon. It's at the back of the ankle, just above the heel, and seems to want to cause trouble for athletes. Although it is said to be not strictly necessary for walkers, it's probably a good idea to stretch out your own Achilles' tendons. Calf muscles can tighten up especially in people with sedentary jobs and lives. You can even stretch both tendons at the same time. Just stand three or four foot-lengths away from a tree or lamppost, and using it for support, lean forward with heels on the ground, bending your knees a bit, until you feel a stretch in your Achilles' tendons. Hold it long enough to feel the tendons and calves relaxing. When you stretch, it's important not to use a bouncing technique, called "ballistic" stretching. Instead of stretching and relaxing the muscles and tendons, ballistic stretching actually makes them tighter because the rhythmical stretch-contraction cycle triggers a protective muscle-tightening reflex in the involved muscle fibers. What is needed for the best stretch is steady extension of a warmed-up muscle.

Another stretch for the Achilles tendon is to stand with the ball of one foot up on a low curbstone and the heel on the street surface leaning forward with knee bent until you feel a stretch in your calf and in the back of your ankle.

To stretch the groin muscles, semi-squat with knees bent and your feet spread almost as wide as you can reach (Squat enough to place your lower legs at right angles to your thighs), now lean to the right side, placing your hands down onto your bent right leg. Your left leg will begin to straighten, and the inner thigh and groin muscles of that leg will be placed on a stretch. Keep your left foot pointed straight ahead, the right one wherever it is comfortable. Then switch sides. Hold each side until you feel your inner thigh and groin muscles not only stretching, out but beginning to let go (relax). No leaning on your knee though; it puts unnatural pressures on the knee joint cartilage. Rest your hand on your thigh. If you need to, hold on to something for support.

This is an important stretch, for our groin muscles can become tight from the limitations we place on our general activities as we get older, so that the possibility of a groin muscle strain or sprain is increased. Groin pulls can be very painful, and can cause disability for an extended period. Sitting on the floor Indian-style (knees bent, legs crossed in front of you) while watching TV will also gently stretch out the groin muscles. For a better stretch, see if you can place the soles of your feet together and allow your knees to fall down toward the floor while you're sitting there Indian-style. Remember that stretching is safer and more effective with a warmed-up muscle, so do not be too enthusiastic here, lest instead of stretching the groin muscles you strain them.

Improving Posture

People ask me about holding in their stomach as they walk, in an effort to strengthen the abdominal wall, and improve their posture. It does help, but I have found that it is difficult to give it the prolonged attention it needs if it is to become an unconscious habit. A minute after you suck it up you are distracted by something, and out it goes again. Then, *if* you remember again as you continue on, you might repeat the effort, but again, you are soon distracted. Notice I used the word "habit" again. That's because people who have good posture, and a modestly flat abdomen, have developed it into a habit over the years. It's not usually the result of physical conditioning alone, unless you're willing to develop six-pack abs by engaging in a strenuous exercise program. Buying a magic machine on TV won't help either. It is really more practical to develop good posture to the point where it becomes an ingrained and unconscious habit—that semi-automatic-pilot we talked about. Of course the best way to have unconscious good posture throughout life is to have had parents who nagged you about it in childhood. But there's hope for the rest of us too, in perseverance and self-discipline, which, after all, is probably exactly what our parents were getting at in the first place, in addition to wanting us to have the sense of well-being and confidence that good posture imparts.

How to do it

Here is a walking trick that really helps. As you hustle along your route, pull in your gut, and tell yourself you will hold it just until you reach that next telephone pole, or the fire hydrant thirty or forty paces ahead. Keep it in your mind for that short distance, then let go. After a time, repeat it. A variation is to hold your stomach in while you count fifty paces, or however many you can without losing your concentration. Make it a game. If you can hold it in for fifty paces, can you hold it in for sixty? As with all such activities, it will eventually become semi-automatic and you'll find yourself standing straighter and taller all the time. Incidentally, if you really pull your abdomen in hard during those brief periods—actually make it hollow, it will strengthen your abdominal muscles significantly, and accelerate the process of obtaining full-time good posture.

Incidentally, as long as we are on the subject of how to improve posture, think about holding in your abdomen and standing taller when engaged in other activities—the entire time it takes to make a cup of tea or to brush your teeth, descend or ascend the stairs, etc. Think up your own. After a time you'll find that you are standing straighter all the time.

Chapter summary; things to think about

Just how good is walking as an exercise?
Why it is very good, and in what specific ways it helps
What kind of walking are we talking about?
What is fast walking?
Stairs, escalators, and parking the car
Doing it in the city
Doing it in the country
Making a route
Walking partners
Dressing for the weather—and to be seen
Counting your pulse: why?
Heart's stroke volume, resting pulse rate
Stretching for safety
Strengthening abdominals—helpful hints
How to improve your posture

17

More on Bones & Joints. Osteoporosis

Why we lose bone mass; osteoporosis

The structure and strength of bones are very much influenced by exercise. Two types of cells unique to bone, osteoblasts and osteoclasts, build up or tear down bone mass in response to need. An easy way to think about it is that osteoblasts build up bone when bone needs to be stronger. Osteoclasts break down bone when the body needs calcium and dietary amounts are insufficient.

In the first case, the building up of bone mass and density is chiefly a response to exercise and adequate calcium in the diet. All exercise places stress on bones, because all of the body's muscles are attached to bone on both ends, by their tendons. The amount of stress placed on the bone depends on the type and duration of the exercise activity. On the other side, reduced bone density and bone strength are common in older people, who do not consume adequate dietary or supplemental calcium and who, because of inactivity, place little if any stress on the bones of their extremities, hips, shoulders, and spine. For reasons related to hormonal differences between men and women, loss of bone mass is more common in women than it is in men.

What to do about it

By increasing exercise levels, and eating more calcium-rich foods, or taking calcium supplements, it's possible for early osteoporosis to be halted, and actually even reversed. Getting out into the sunshine causes the skin to produce vitamin D, which is necessary for the absorption of dietary calcium. In addition to the usual admonitions to drink more milk, and eat more cooked greens, in the section on food and diet I will tell you a way to wring the last gram of calcium out of home-prepared soups, broth, and stews.

Through the eons, mankind's diet has changed, and we are much less physically active than our forebears were. For most of us, today's occupations and life-styles simply do not provide many opportunities for the type of manual labor that places stress on bones. This is one of the reasons that dietary calcium supplements are recommended. Calcium is rather difficult to digest, and the jury is still out on which calcium compound is absorbed in greatest quantity, but calcium citrate seems to head the list at the present time. It's available in 300 mg pills and capsules, which usually also contain a small quantity of magnesium. Capsules are easier to swallow, and are a bit easier to absorb than the pill form. Four a day is the recommended amount, usually two before or with breakfast, and two more at dinnertime.

The Appendix of this book contains a short list of calcium-rich foods. A few foods are antagonistic to calcium absorption, but I wouldn't worry too much about them. If you are diligent in all the other things you ought to be concentrating on, like exercising, walking, and insofar as your diabetic or weight-control diet will allow, eating calcium-rich foods, then you shouldn't be worried about whether or not you can have that extra cup of coffee.

Even non-strenuous exercises improve bone mass. As your stamina and general fitness improve, it is beneficial during your walking or workouts to push yourself a little, beyond your attained exercise limits, because bones grow accustomed to the same level of activity and will not

continue to strengthen. It is the added stress of pushing it a
bit that strengthens them, and increases their mass. But
please do not, in your enthusiasm, test your limits in the
beginning. That's not fair to your newly active body.

In older people, strengthening exercises are important,
to reduce the risk of falling, which can cause fractures,
especially in the more porous bones of old age. The
improved leg-strength, and increased bone density, that
come with an active life-style, afford better balance, so the
likelihood of falling is reduced. And if an accident does
occur, the chance of suffering a fracture is lessened.

Aerobic exercise helps to stabilize and support the
joints, and even reduces inflammation in joints. If you are
troubled by early arthritis, bicycling and fast walking are
very beneficial. Swimming and exercising in water are also
good exercise modalities.

Most doctors I know encourage arthritis patients to
engage in strengthening exercises as a first treatment, even
before prescribing pain relievers. Patients who rely on pain-
killing drugs from the outset may overuse and abuse their
knees, which do not have strong supportive muscle tissue to
protect them from damage.

Joints require motion to stay healthy. Long periods of
inactivity cause older people's joints to stiffen, and the
adjoining tissues to atrophy. An exercise program that
includes low-impact aerobics and strength training has
benefits for osteo-arthritic patients as well as for diabetics.

Two Common Types of Arthritis

As opposed to rheumatoid arthritis, which is primarily
inflammatory, and characterized by inflammation of the
synovial membrane of joints, osteoarthritis is a form of
arthritis caused by degenerative thinning and loss of joint
cartilage. Although inflammation can, and usually does
ensue with advanced degeneration of the joint cartilages, the
genesis of osteoarthritis is not inflammatory. With aging, the
water content of joint cartilage increases and the protein

makeup of cartilage degenerates. Over the years, repetitive use of the joints irritates and inflames the cartilage, causing the typical joint pain and swelling.

Eventually, joint cartilage begins to degenerate by flaking, or developing tiny crevasses in the bearing surfaces. Loss of the cartilage cushion in the joint then causes friction between the bones, leading to pain, and limitation of joint mobility. The inflammation of the cartilage can also stimulate new bone outgrowths (spurs) to form in and around the joints. How can one justify exercising in the presence of this condition? Read on.

Glucosamine and Chondroitin

Glucosamine and chondroitin sulfate supplements are now recommended by many doctors to help restore lost cartilage in joints. The combination is available without prescription in vitamin stores and pharmacies, and daily dosages are listed on the label.

Investigators at the National Institutes of Health have been looking into whether glucosamine and chondroitin sulfate can actually improve and protect the quality of the cartilage in joints affected by osteoarthritis, because animal studies with a radioactive tracer attached to the compound have shown its presence in joints after ingestion.

In general, arthritis patients who embark on exercise programs report less disability and pain, and are able to perform daily chores and remain independent longer than their inactive peers. As well, regular range-of-motion exercises will increase the limits of movement (range) in a joint or muscle. Good examples are Yoga and Tai Chi, which focus on flexibility, balance, and proper breathing. As with brisk walking, these activities also lower stress levels, help to reduce blood pressure, and have significant beneficial effects on cholesterol levels. Every sunny morning in our little Upper East Side park, Tai Chi people can be seen doing their serene, slow ballet.

Caveats and Encouragements

As with every wonderful activity in life, there are a few caveats. Temper your enthusiasm with common sense. Don't overdo in the beginning. Listen to your body. A good rule for the first few months is to quit while you are still wanting more. This is not only a safety mechanism. It will help maintain your enthusiasm for tomorrow's walk or work-out. If those joint pains don't disappear with walking and stretching, make a visit to your doctor, or let a physical therapist have a look before resuming your walks. Do not allow it to become a deterrent, though. It's all too easy to slip into the couch potato mode when we are faced with difficulties.

It's important to understand that if you become lightheaded, dizzy, short of breath, or feel an irregular, or rapid heartbeat, or have chest pain, or even if your pulse rate does not come back down to normal within a few minutes of stopping exercise, you should desist, and consult your doctor before resuming.

Okay, it's frustrating. Just when you were getting enthusiastic, you have to postpone your walking. I remind you that the goal is worth it. Remember? Lower LDL, higher HDL, more stable blood sugar levels, increased stamina and energy, stronger legs, a stronger heart with lessened risk of heart attack, lower blood pressure, better balance, a clearer head? I have found that as we get older, nothing destroys self-confidence more than weakness in the legs, and inability to walk briskly. It makes us feel old, and out of the mainstream of activities. When you look at old people shuffling along, and barely able to climb the steps into the local bus, it's easy to understand their expression of surrender. They have been defeated and they know it. Sad. And for a significant number of them, unnecessary.

Chapter summary; things to think about

Osteoblasts and osteoclasts and what they do
Osteoporosis defined
Preventing osteoporosis
Exercise; benefits to bones
Diet and calcium supplements
Leg strength and falling
Early treatment for arthritis
Glucosamine and Chondroitin sulfate
Hope for the weakening legs of the aged
A Caveat
Maintaining enthusiasm despite set-backs

18

The Truth About Getting a better figure

Snake Oil

In today's world of sophisticated advertising and easy communication via television, the internet, and print media, it is easy to find yourself believing promises of six-pack abs, tight buns, and Playboy thighs. The beautiful girls and guys are standing by the machine to prove that it works.

But promises that you can selectively lose weight in certain areas of the body are mostly snake oil. Exercising your abdomen by doing sit ups, or simulating them on a machine, will indeed result in stronger abdominal muscles, but—and this is a big but—you cannot burn away abdominal fat or thigh fat selectively. If your abdomen becomes flatter because of these exercises, it is because you have strengthened the underlying muscular wall and at the same time reduced general body fat by means of the exercise activity, a fine ambition in and of itself, but you have to understand what is actually happening.

Using a stair-climbing machine will reduce the fat in your buttocks only insofar as the exercise itself is aerobic and your muscles begin to seek energy sources via the Krebs cycle. When that happens, the Krebs cycle doesn't just select out the fat that overlies the muscles you are exercising. The Krebs cycle is an equal-opportunity fuel provider. Fat is mobilized from all fat-storage depots throughout the body at the same time, internal fat as well as sub-cutaneous fat and other visible fat. Of course, as the underlying gluteal and thigh muscles become toned and strengthened from the exercise, they assume a more pleasing profile.

So don't let the hucksters fool you. And don't fool yourself either. Thunder thighs will not selectively be reduced in size and fat content by strengthening them on a machine marketed for that purpose, but they will be reduced in size, and strengthened by monitoring food choices and getting serious about aerobic exercising. Instead of doing only thigh-strengthening exercises on a weight machine, let that be just a part of your overall program. Get yourself on a treadmill or stationary bicycle four or five times a week, and each time you do, stay on it until you have burned up all the quickly-available glucose floating around in the blood stream and large muscles and the Krebs cycle has a chance to kick in and begin to burn body fat. You know now that depending on the level of the particular activity, it takes variably fifteen minutes to half an hour before the Krebs cycle starts to seek out general body fat for its fuel (In part, the lead-time depends on when and what you ate). After thirty minutes on the treadmill, you can, if you want, get on that stair-climber to further strengthen and reshape your gluteal and thigh muscles.

I don't want to take away what I've just emphasized, but I want you to know that weight lifting and resistance training of the type seen on television commercials for exercise machines does indeed burn body fat, but it's important to understand that it happens in response to programmatic, progressive weight training, supplemented by a vigorous aerobics program. Off-camera, the people demonstrating those exercise machines on television are engaged in just that. They run, they swim, they walk. That's why they look so fit.

For our purposes, taking into account our needs, our

present physical condition and age, aerobic exercise with a little strength training added into the mix is without question the better way to go. And if you're not fit enough or young enough for weight training, that's okay too. Fast walking will accomplish our goals splendidly.

How Much and How Long?

Every week there is another expert on television or in print with a theory on how much, and what kind of exercise we should do. There are suggestions for programs to maintain your weight at its present level, programs for slimming down, building endurance, developing muscle strength, and on and on. Some suggest exercising three times a week, others suggest every other day (it's difficult to set up an easy-to-remember weekly schedule with this schedule).

Still other experts maintain that you must exercise every day, one day aerobic, the next day weight training. If that's not enough confusion, opinion is divided on whether the workout should be one hour, two hours, or just a half hour. It's enough to make you wish it would all just go away. Which, unfortunately for many of us, it does—just as soon as we switch on the TV or go into the kitchen for a snack.

My suggestion is to forget all of it. At this point, unless you have decided to engage a trainer at a gym, what is needed most of all, is to get up off the sofa four or five times a week and onto a treadmill or out on the sidewalks or roads, walking fast for a half an hour. Skip a day in between if you want, but if you feel you are capable of walking every day and are comfortable doing it, that's perfectly all right too. If sticking to your full route or circuit on consecutive days seems too tiring, shorten up a bit, or walk slower on the second of the two days. That's enough for starters. Before long, your body will tell you that you need more activity, and by then you will be enthusiastic enough to delve into all the theories without confusing yourself. At that point, and depending on your age, you might review the sections in this book on the Krebs cycle, and decide how you can reduce body fat even more rapidly with weight training added into your aerobic exercise routine.

If your three or four times a week walks aren't enough, you might then want to think about doing your full route every day. At a fast military pace, it's possible to cover two miles in about thirty minutes, as I do. Thirty to thirty-three minutes will do it, and that is a very small slice out of your day. Try to set it up for early mornings. You will be more energetic for the rest of the day, and you will enjoy the day more knowing that you have done it.

Never allow the theories to disable your will and your early efforts along with it. This is the danger of trying to decide at the beginning which program is best. It's too much too soon. It overloads the circuits, and the indecision leads to inaction. Just make the simple decision to walk three times a week and maybe once on the weekend, (to make up for those inevitable rainy days when you have to stay indoors and step up and down on the bottom step of your staircase). Gradually build your distance and speed. And when you feel up to it, and you are enthusiastic about doing more, add some simple muscle-building routines on the in-between days, as described in this book. Or, as I mentioned above, just do your walk every day. And please remember how important it is to persist in those first efforts until that habit kicks in.

Pulse monitoring on a treadmill

If you choose the treadmill route, you will be pleased to know that most treadmills monitor your pulse rate, either through the machine's handholds or via your own monitor, if you have one. After hanging on to the sweaty handholds for a couple of months, I broke down and bought a pulse monitor at a sporting goods store. Like most of us, after a few weeks on the treadmill, you will want to swing your arms freely for a better workout, and you can't do that if you have to hang on to the hand bar to see your pulse rate.

Besides, it's more fun to swing your arms, and you can actually accelerate your heart rate to some degree by swinging your arms for a few minutes, then resting them on the machine's hand-holds to slow down your pulse-rate.

At my present state of fitness, whether or not I swing my arms on the treadmill makes a difference of about 6 beats a minute in my pulse. Of course you can slow down or speed up the treadmill, or regulate the degree of slope to accomplish the same thing, but I take my fun where I find it. It's interesting to see how large an effect a small thing like swinging or not swinging your arms has, and it provides a more immediate way to increase or decrease your heart rate than changing the speed or slope of the treadmill.

When I use the pulse monitor that I bought, I fasten the sender around my chest with the elastic band provided (the sender is built right in to the plastic band and the whole thing is washable), then I slip on the wrist watch which picks up the signal. The one I bought is made by Polar™, which turned out to be the company that provided the pulse counter in the treadmills where I work out, so my pulse rate shows up on the treadmill's 'dashboard' as well as on my wristwatch.

I chose the cheapest model. It has more than enough features and readouts to inform and confuse you. It displays instantaneous pulse rate, an elapsed time display divided into ten-minute segments, and at the end of the session, it tells you your average heart rate over the entire time of the session, and how long you exercised. The little rig is great for walking outdoors too. They are inexpensive, and easy to find at major sporting goods stores.

Chapter summary; things to think about

Losing weight in the real world
Selective, localized weight loss is a myth
The Krebs Cycle again
Making a training schedule
Keeping it simple
Thirty-minute sessions three or four times a week
Best time of day
On the treadmill
Using pulse monitors so you can swing your arms on
 the treadmill
How they work
Cheaper is just as good if not better
What the pulse monitor tells you

19

Weight Lifting On The Cheap

Stretch bands as a substitute for weights

I want to tell you about an inexpensive, fun way to supplement your walking, a way to tone and develop the large muscles in the upper part of your body to complement the increasing strength in your legs. It provides the same workout as lifting weights does, but you do not have to buy dumbbells and barbells, or even go to a gym to do it. Instead, you use elastic bands—large stretchable bands especially designed for the purpose. They are thin rubber straps about six feet long and five to six inches wide. There are several brands available.

The one that I am familiar with is "Thera-Band". When stretched, provide resistance similar to that of lifting weights. The strips vary in thickness to provide more or less resistance and are color coded; yellow for easy, red for medium effort, and green for more resistance. If these become too easy over time, stronger bands are available. The nice thing about them is that you can also customize their strength and resistance by shortening up on an individual band as you become stronger.

Exercise bands are available in rolls from which lengths

are cut, and are also available in boxes of three bands each, graduated in resistance. Boxed sets of three cost about $12.00, and they are available in most sporting goods stores. Some hospital supply stores and pharmacies stock the bands in long rolls, and will cut five or six-foot lengths for you. I recently found rolls of several different strengths at a hospital supply store, priced at about a dollar per foot.

As you might expect, the boxed sets are also available on the internet in the inexpensive range of about three to five dollars a box, but shipping charges might cost more than the product itself.

Stretch bands are surprisingly versatile. The bands themselves take up very little space, and can be kept handy for use in any room of the house. If you buy the boxed set of three, it comes with illustrated instructions for several exercises. For example, if you hold the ends of the band in your hands and step down on the center of the band with one or both feet, you can do regular arm curls. Start with ten or fifteen repetitions. Rest thirty seconds or so, and do a second set.

A second simple exercise is to wrap the band around each hand out in front of your chest, leaving about one foot or a little more of band between. Holding both arms straight out in front of you, slowly separate your arms until they are out to the sides at shoulder level and the band is stretched against your chest. Then slowly bring your arms back to the original position. Try for ten reps, and repeat the set as you did for the arm curls. Always exhale on the extension or pull, and inhale coming back. Do not hold your breath (it raises blood pressure). If you have difficulty timing your breathing to coincide with stretching and relaxing the band, count each repetition on the stretch part of the cycle out loud, either from one to ten or from ten down to zero. This will assure that you are exhaling on the lift.

These are just two of many exercises. You can simulate practically every barbell or dumbbell exercise with stretch bands. Just to give you a start, here are a few in easy-to-follow form.

Biceps (arm) Curl

Stand with ends of band in hands, arms at sides, right foot (or both feet) over loop of band.
Flex forearms upward and return hands slowly to their relaxed positions.
Exhale on lift. Count aloud on lift if needed.
Aim for ten or fifteen repetitions, then rest and swing arms about to loosen muscles.

Deltoid Lift

Stand with ends of band in hands, arms at your sides, loop of band under both feet.
Slowly lift arms out away from body sideways. Do not try to lift arms as high as shoulders.
Slowly lower arms to sides.
Exhale up, inhale down.
Ten reps, rest and jiggle arms, then ten more.

Shoulder Shrug

Stand with hands at sides, band looped under both feet, holding band on a tight stretch.
Shrug shoulders fifteen times.
Rest, then roll shoulders five or six times toward back and then do the same number of times toward front.
Do a second set if you feel up to it but do *not* over-do. There is no need to prove how strong or fit you are. The name of the game is increasing your fitness, not testing your strength or your limits.
For more resistance, shorten up on band.

Triceps Toning (back of upper arm)

Wrap band around left hand and hold it tight to upper part of chest close to centerline. Wrap band around other hand about six inches in front of left hand.

Holding left hand firmly to chest, slowly move right hand away until right arm is straight out in front of you. If the resistance is not enough, start with hands closer together.
Ten to fifteen reps, rest and jiggle, then ten more.
Repeat with left arm, reversing hands.

Alternate Method Deltoid Lift

Hold band by ends, stepping on the center of the band. Secure one end of band with left hand and keep that arm at side throughout.
Holding other end of band with right hand, slowly lift right arm away from body sideways keeping arm reasonably straight; no higher than shoulder.
Lower slowly. Repeat. Change sides. When you step on the band for this exercise, allow a little more band on the lifting side.
To double the benefit with any weight exercise, including stretch bands, lower as slowly as you lift, the slower the better, in both directions.

Back Stretcher & Triceps Toner

Step on end of band with heel.
Hold other end of band with both hands behind head about level with ears. (Hands are placed as though you were adjusting the back of your shirt collar.)
Slowly lift arms up until arms are straight up above your head.
Lower slowly.
This is a strenuous exercise; start with only a few reps.
Rest and jiggle your arms between sets.

Improving insulin sensitivity with weight training

With all of the above exercises, increase the number of repetitions and sets as you feel you are able. I may not have stressed this in the section on insulin, but it has been shown that in addition to weight training, regular aerobic exercise, even of moderate intensity, improves insulin sensitivity. I am not referring here to the reactivation of glucose receptors. That only occurs by exercising a muscle to the point of fatigue during very strenuous weight lifting. The mechanism I'm talking about here is that which comes about because of the changes in our metabolism during and after aerobic exercise. The regular physical activity burns away blood sugar before great quantities of insulin have to be released to change it into fat and triglycerides (blood fats).

By now you know that moderate, regular exercise helps to protect the heart in people with Type II diabetes even if they have no risk factors for heart disease other than the diabetes itself. Exercise helps replace sedentary habits that usually lead to snacking. It has also been suggested that exercise itself may even act as a mild appetite suppressant. Isn't that a nice little extra benefit?

NOTE: Although weight training is excellent for maintaining and improving strength, it cannot be counted on as a weight-loss method unless the lifter is an enthusiast, and carefully monitors food intake as well. For the older person it won't build cardiac muscle and stamina as well as aerobics do, but added to an aerobics program it is a wonderful way to maintain upper body strength. Think about trying stretch bands on your in-between days.

Chapter summary; things to think about

Weight training with Elastic Bands
Color Coding and resistance levels
Where to buy them
How they are used.
Some exercises explained
How exercise reduces insulin output and lowers
 blood sugar
Exercise as an appetite suppressant

20

Nourishment

The necessary ingredient that most diet plans lack

We see new diet books coming out all the time. And among the promises and stories of amazing weight loss over short periods of time, I hear tales of people in trouble—loss of energy, feelings of weakness, dizziness, nausea, blood cholesterol and/or plasma sugar levels going through the roof, and so on. If you take a look at the hundreds of diet books in your local bookstore, you will realize that dieting by the book is an utter failure. Seeing a "satisfied user" on TV saying, "It's the best diet I've ever been on!" gives the game away, doesn't it? I've heard this more times than I can remember, directly from people I know. I always wonder, if a diet plan is so wonderful why is it necessary to compare it to other past diets, or even to have to go on other diets? Why, in fact, should there need to be a wonderful new diet plan every month or two?

The reason is simple, though not too obvious. It's because most, if not all of them, do not provide the one indispensable ingredient without which a diet is doomed to failure.

In addition to providing sensible food choices, a diet plan must provide a means of changing your attitude toward the role that food should play in your life, which is of course, nourishment, fuel for the machine. Not solace, comfort, or a substitute for love.

And then of course, a little closer to home, there's my own little tale of woe, yet another good example of best intentions gone awry, this time with life-threatening consequences.

So let's get it straight here and now; you shouldn't starve yourself, you shouldn't restrict yourself to all protein, no protein, all meat, no meat, all carbohydrates, no carbohydrates, all vegetables, no vegetables. Nourishment means just that; giving your body what it needs to function.

To that, may I add the words, "at its best"? This means supplying the right amount and types of nutrients to energize you, to rebuild your body as it suffers daily wear and tear, and to help maintain its resistance to disease. What is needed? Amino acids as provided by quality protein, carbohydrates, vitamins and minerals, and fiber (or roughage, as it used to be called), and small amounts of the right kind of fats. What foods will I be suggesting?

What to eat

Let's get specific. This is where we're headed; rough-cut oatmeal, Nabisco Shredded Wheat and Bran, skim milk, egg whites from packages or directly from eggs, everything that swims, most shellfish and crustaceans like lobster, crabs, and shrimp (see note below), all green leafy vegetables (including ones not commonly prepared, such as kale, mustard greens, rob broccoli, escarole, collard greens—all delicious!), all the squashes (butternut, acorn, crookneck, spaghetti squash, summer squash, winter squash, zucchini), tomatoes, bell peppers, beans of all descriptions, fruits and berries in small quantities, no-fat dairy products (no-fat cheeses, skim milk, the new, olive oil margarines; Olivio), and of course, all of the "free" foods mentioned throughout this book, as well as small quantities of nuts.

I left out meats didn't I? It is difficult to find meats that are low enough in fats to help you get and stay healthy, but we'll include some along the way.

When it comes to cholesterol, lobster and shrimp have an undeserved bad reputation. A serving of seven large shrimp contains 78 milligrams of cholesterol, the same amount of lobster has 61 milligrams, but they are rich in omega 3 fatty acids, minerals, and vitamins like folic acid, vitamin A, and retinol (an antioxidant related to vitamin A which is found in green and yellow vegetables, egg yolk, and fish-liver oil). Small quantities of these crustaceans add variety, and are excellent sources of these minerals and vitamins.

What NOT to eat

What else have I left out? The following *won't* be included later: most deli meats and cheeses, frankfurters, ribs and sausages of all types, all commercial fast foods (burgers, fries, shakes, breaded chicken nuggets, etc. All chips, (all means *all*) dips, and deep-fried treats, frozen dinners of any stripe, no matter what they promise, breads, bagels, cake, corn muffins and bran muffins (one commercial corn muffin contains more saturated fat than two eggs! . . .to say nothing of trans fats), English muffins, packaged and packaged single-portion cakey stuff like Twinkies, Devil Dogs, jelly doughnuts, etc.

Adults, and kids as well, will live healthier, longer lives without them. Don't allow your kids or grandchildren to get started on them, and in addition to the immediate benefits, the children won't carry the bad habit into adulthood with them—what we used to call having a "sweet tooth", when I was a kid.

While not in fact poisons, for any diabetic, heart patient, or person fighting a weight problem, most of the above foods should be considered as toxic, if only in the interests of modifying our attitude toward them. In the dictionary, the word "poison" is defined as a substance that causes injury, illness or death, especially by chemical means.

Over the long term, isn't that exactly what these foods do? If we're to win this battle for a healthier, longer life, we need all the support we can muster. It is even *more* important for people with a weight problem to take this to heart.

Little-known dietary Tips

In addition to small amounts of whole wheat or barley added to broths, millet is an excellent grain for older people because it contains silica, which helps to keep bones supple.

Plant foods boost calcium and other minerals in your body. Calcium tip: Make home-made stock with bones, seafood shells or vegetable scraps, all excellent sources of minerals. Adding a tiny amount of vinegar (a capful) or wine (a two-ounce shot glass) to the stock while it simmers will draw calcium out of the bones or seafood shells and into the broth where it becomes available to ingest.

One more thing; forget about those protein drinks that are touted as weight-loss aids—you know, the ones you see the beautiful girls and guys drinking on television? Touted as high in necessary proteins, low in calories? *Recent studies have shown that we actually eat more when we include them in our diets.* The reason is that we are hungry again in one or two hours. Tests showed that people who drink these shakes actually gained weight! The old Chinese meal syndrome again.

Finding the holes in your diet

One final dietary tip, and it's a gem. I call it "finding the holes in your diet". Essentially, it means that we cannot merely adjust our intake of the main items in our daily menus and congratulate ourselves on a job well done. Very possibly, there is a hidden enemy someplace, very likely more than one; I'm thinking of a condiment loaded with sugar or fat or fatty acids, a once-a-week dessert indulgence, a box of buttered popcorn at the movies, a handful of salty or sweet treats as we pass by the kitchen, a beer or two with the fellows. The strategy should be, that until we understand the consequences of even a single pretzel, we should find out the carbohydrate content of *every last thing* that passes our lips.

Case in Point

I have a friend who put himself on an Atkins type diet —we all know what that is so I won't elaborate—and he's wondering why he is not losing weight. When he asked me about it, I suggested that he make a complete-to-the-last-item list of *everything* that he ate and drank over a two week period. When I constructed a data base of his intake I discovered that he was eating upwards of 200 grams of carbohydrate a day. He didn't realize, for example, that by switching from blueberries to fresh strawberries on his breakfast cereal he could reduce his daily carbohydrate intake by ten grams, because compared by weight, strawberries contain one gram and blueberries have eleven grams of carbohydrates. Or that a slice of whole wheat Italian bread has 31 grams of carbohydrate as compared to a slice of Italian white, which has 21 grams. His entire diet was riddled with similar poor choices.

That's exactly what I mean by 'finding the holes in your diet'. When we begin to diet, it doesn't usually occur to us to count the incidentals—the toppings, the bottled salad dressings, the sodas, the crackers, the peanuts, the chips.

I must tell you from my own experience with patients (and with myself), that we actually *want* not to notice these small dietary transgressions, so that we can indulge without feeling that we've broken our diet.

While mild lapses may be all right after you've gotten your weight down to where you want it to be, and you're deep into the active lifestyle, avoiding these little overlooked indulgences can very possibly prevent you from getting there in the first place.

So find the holes in your diet and eliminate them. If none are immediately evident and you are not losing weight, make a detailed list on paper of everything you put into your mouth over two or three weeks time—every last thing. Then buy a paperback book that lists carbohydrate content of foods and tally them up. I'm betting you will be surprised at what you will discover.

Chapter summary; things to think about

Quick weight-loss diets; do they work?
What kind of a diet should we eat?
Foods to eat and foods not to eat
Some foods are poisons for the diabetic
Nutrition Tips
A simple way to increase calcium intake
Finding the "holes" in your diet
Keep a record of everything you eat to discover the holes in your diet, and be prepared for a surprise.

21

Meal choices—a start in the right direction

Recipe books vs. doing it yourself

Here are some ideas for low-carbohydrate, nourishing meals which, with the help of my S.O., I worked out for our own needs. Hopefully, they will serve to get you thinking, and start you on the right path. I do not believe that books full of recipes written by other people are very useful in the long run. For one thing, they take the decisions and the thinking out of your hands. Doing the analyses yourself, and then working out safe, tasty recipes, are important parts of your metamorphosis.

Also, because you did not participate in their development, most of the recipes in magazines and books are soon forgotten, and replaced by others, copied or cut out of yet other magazines and cook books. And here's the kicker—more often than not, the new replacements are reversions back toward comfort foods.

Start instead, by buying a small loose leaf notebook to record your own recipes in, and begin to make up your own meal plans and safe snacking foods. Think them through yourself.

A Breakfast Omelet – one of many possibilities

For breakfast, I usually have egg whites, either separated by me or purchased in a carton. A little more expensive, the commercial brands are pure, contain over 99% pure egg whites, are fat-free, and practically devoid of carbohydrates. One container has only 30 calories. The recipe is simplicity itself. I start with some sliced-up fresh tomato in a non-stick pan, pour the Egg Beaters or your own separated egg whites over it and when it's nearly cooked, add a cut-up slice of no-fat cheese—any "flavor" will do; "American", cheddar, Swiss—they all taste the same. Flip one half over the other like a half-moon, and turn off the flame. That's it. You can add raw or cooked spinach, mushrooms, left over broccoli or cauliflower florets, chopped up onion or other veggies, as long as they're not the starchy kind. And just forget about the fried potatoes.

As you might remember from the earlier chapters, I eat it either alone or with a Wasa bread and a cup of tea or coffee.

Speaking of coffee, I have discovered a delicious coffee substitute for those who want to, or must, give up caffeine completely, including the not-inconsiderable amount remaining in "decaffeinated" coffee. The product is called CAFIX, made in Switzerland of grains, chicory, and (of all things!) figs and beet root. A heaping teaspoon of the powder in a big mug, with boiling water poured over it, makes a dark, tasty, foamy cup of "coffee". Essentially free of carbs, it can be drunk black or with milk (and carbohydrates!). The label suggests that a creamy latte' can be made by pouring steaming hot milk over the Cafix instead of water, but I do not recommend it because of the carbs.

If you can't stand the temptation, get out of the kitchen

After I eat my omelet, I leave the kitchen. You should

too. I learned from experience, that breakfast time conversations over that extra cup of coffee almost invariably lead to munching on comfort foods, often on a "just-this-once-won't-hurt" basis, and is more likely to occur if someone else is having something with their coffee.

Oscar Wilde said it perfectly. "I can resist anything except temptation." You will be healthier and thinner if you don't put yourself in the way of temptation to begin with.

For Cereal Lovers (or egg haters)

There are only two cereals to consider. You would be wise to look upon the rest as inedible, no matter what they claim on TV, or on the box, about the good taste, percentages of daily requirements, and amounts of vitamins in them. Although some are rich in fiber, they all contain sugar in great quantity. Many contain preservatives and artificial color. In other words, for a diabetic, or a person fighting to get thin, they're poison. Never touch them. The only way to do that is to not buy them. If you don't have them in the house, you can't be tempted.

Have you gotten a look at commercial dog and cat foods recently? Multi-colored pellets full of artificial colorings and loaded with salt. (I tasted one.) Dogs are color-blind for Heaven's sake! Of course the dog doesn't control the purse strings, but if he did, I bet he wouldn't spend his money on that stuff.

And you don't have to buy those sugar-laden cereals for the children either. Buying them for the kids can be a sneaky little rationalization that allows you to eat them once in a while without feeling the guilt associated with buying them for yourself, so watch out! Despite your doubts, the children's complaining will stop, and they will eventually come around to eating the good stuff. And they will be healthier for it. Get the children in the habit of sweetening their cereal with fresh fruits or berries instead of sugar or artificial sweeteners.

The Two and Only

The first of the only two cereals I recommend, is Post's Nabisco Shredded Wheat 'N Bran, and the other, a hot cereal, is old fashioned Quaker Oatmeal. Shredded wheat with bran needs no explanations. It can be eaten plain or with a few berries, or a couple of thin apple or pear slices, and it can be eaten with cold skim mill or with warm skim milk, which softens it. It has become so popular that it is becoming difficult to find on grocers' shelves. Customers are running off with three and four boxes.

I should tell you, that if you haven't tried fat-free milk lately you are in for a pleasant surprise. That watery, faintly blue stuff is long gone. In its place is flavorful, creamy-tasting white milk, abundant in calcium. It's rich enough to use in coffee or tea.

The oatmeal should be Old-Fashioned Quaker Oats, or another plain oatmeal brand. Be sure it's the "old-fashioned" long-cooking variety, not the quick-cooking kind. Old-fashioned oatmeal has a lower glycemic index. The instant variety of oatmeal is simply regular oatmeal ground up finer for quicker cooking. The finer cut also makes it more easily digested, so it raises blood sugar faster and higher than regular, rough-cut oatmeal. If you choose a brand other than Quaker, be sure the ingredients list includes only "rolled oats", and nothing else.

You do not have to cook oatmeal for the recommended time. If it's hot and soft, that's good enough—nothing like the five to seven minutes suggested on the box. You can cook it for perhaps two or three minutes, tops. Less digestible? A little, but less digestible means that intestinal transport is faster, which is better for your blood sugar because less is digested and absorbed. It also provides more roughage (fiber). Your alimentary canal will absorb out the B-vitamins, phosphorus, and potassium anyway. Serve oatmeal the same as the shredded wheat; plain, or with berries, apple, etc.

If you absolutely, positively cannot live without

sweetening it, use Splenda. It's chemical-free and has no after-taste. But try to wean yourself. Remember how sugar conditions your taste buds to want more? Well, artificial sweeteners do the same thing. I no longer use sweetener in or on anything. I've come to prefer coffee, tea, cereals and such without it. If my host or hostess serves me sweetened coffee by mistake I can't get it down. I go into my S.O.'s mode of politely holding the cup but not putting it up to my lips. And I smile a lot, like she does.

Lunch

Here are two or three nourishing lunches to tide you over until dinner. One is "Tom's Tuna Tsalad" as my friend Phil dubbed it, and the other is another, as-yet-unnamed tuna salad. If you like, you can name it after the pounds you'll lose. How about, "Pounds away salad"?

Tom's Tuna Tsalad

I wash and slice up one or two stalks of celery, leaves and all, and a wedge of dill pickle, and throw them into a bowl with a few sliced almonds or cracked walnut meats. I add a can of drained, solid-pack light tuna packed in water, and a small dollop of low-fat mayo. I try to have more celery than tuna. It is not the sort of tuna salad that restaurants serve—which looks to me like it is nearly all tuna with mayonnaise in it. Make sure yours contains a much greater proportion of celery and pickle than tuna. It tastes better, anyway.

If low-fat mayonnaise troubles you in terms of the fat involved, a little extra-virgin olive oil, and either vinegar or the juice of half a lemon make an equally good-tasting dressing for tuna salad. Sometimes when I use this dressing, I add a few grape tomatoes cut in half.

Buy the best light tuna. Don't go for the cheaper dark stuff, which contains less of the monounsaturated oils that lower LDL cholesterol. Besides, you deserve the best. You've worked hard all your life, and how many more times will you be passing this way?

The tuna salad is simple, nourishing, and quick. It is usually too much to eat, but it can be saved in the fridge or shared. It is important to remember that as nourishing as they are, nuts are fatty, so go easy. If you hate pickle, leave it out. They should never be "bread and butter" pickles, or any other sugary types, by the way. Read the label. Buy only Jewish dills, half-sours, or garlic dills.

Salad Number Two

I open a can of drained tuna into a cereal bowl and make a dressing of some mustard—enough to give it a little bite—then I add a little extra-virgin olive oil and some vinegar or lemon juice, break up the tuna and add it all to a nice bowl of rinsed and drained salad greens. Escarole is my personal favorite, but any green will do. You can add a few almond slices or some cracked walnuts to this one too. Top it off with oregano or basil if you prefer, a little salt and black pepper and share it with your S.O.

While it's true that olive oil raises HDL and lowers LDL cholesterol, it doesn't mean you can throw caution to the wind and pour in half a cup. Also remember that even low-fat mayo is fatty. If you can get past the taste, fat-free mayo is not. (I'd rather not, thank you. I opt instead for extra-virgin olive oil with vinegar or lemon juice.) This might be a good place to mention that balsamic vinegar contains quite a bit of sugar because it is not a vinegar in the ordinary sense; it's made from a reduction of cooked grape juice.

If you count the carbohydrates or calories in the above recipes you will be pleasantly surprised.

Another Fish for Lunch

It is canned salmon. It can be prepared the same as the tuna salad described above, but it is also delicious on a bed of lettuce with fresh lemon juice squeezed on it. It's also great as a light dinner. Again, buy the best salmon. Nothing will discourage you quicker than unappetizing food. We're dealing with your life and health here. And think of all the money you're going to save by not having to buy expensive steaks, chops, and roasts (and sweets!).

A Bean Salad

This is made with a can of chick peas or cannellini, lots of celery with leaves included, a cut-up tomato or some grape tomatoes, oil and vinegar or lemon juice, salt, fresh ground pepper and oregano or basil to suit your taste. Better share this one; despite their importance, beans are high in carbohydrates. To be on the safe side, don't eat bread with it. And be sure to take two hydroxycitric acid caps half-an-hour before you begin preparing it. The extra minutes you allow for the hydroxycitric acid to digest before eating your meal will improve its effect.

The Second-Quickest Lunch

This is simplicity itself. A spoonful of plain, non-fat cottage cheese or ricotta in a cereal bowl, with a couple of spoonfuls of your favorite salsa and some slivered almonds or a couple of walnut meats as garnish. If your physical conditioning is advanced enough, eat it with a Wasa bread. Have an iced or hot tea and be gone. 'Nuff said.

By the way, the winner of the grand prize for the absolutely quickest lunch was mentioned in a previous chapter. It's putting a little mustard on two slices of boiled ham and a slice of your favorite cheese, then rolling it up and eating it, as either finger food or with a knife and fork. You may remember that I suggested that although it seems like a fatty lunch, in comparison to all the meat and cheese in a regular sandwich, the rolled up version is skimpy victuals indeed. And it's important to remember that the carbohydrates in the bread that you're *not* eating in this "sandwich" would raise cholesterol almost as effectively as the meat and cheese. (See Chapter Eight.)

I will be the first to admit that some of these recipes are meager doin's. There's not much variety here. I haven't made an effort to make them colorful, exotic, or even especially appetizing. There's method to my madness. With a couple of exceptions, which I will tell you about, I want to play down the importance of tantalizing, lip-smacking foods in your life, to encourage you to get your mind out of the icebox. In every culture across the world, food preparation has an illustrious history, and great eats are one of mankind's glorious achievements, but in fact, despite all the glamour, attractive and delicious victuals are a big part of what got us to where we are today, a society besieged by obesity, diabetes, unhealthy, overweight kids who lack the energy to use their bodies vigorously, and a maturity beset by health problems.

Chapter summary; things to think about

Why you should make up your own recipes and not
 get them from books and magazines
Keep a notebook of your favorites
Breakfasts
An omelet
The only two cereals safe to eat; Shredded Wheat 'N
 Bran
Old-fashioned rough-cut oatmeal
Lunches
Two tuna salads
Salmon
A bean salad
The quickest lunches

22

More Food Ideas

Peppers & Onions

Here, in her own words, is Fabiola's recipe for Peppers and Onions.

"I would like to tell you how wonderful this simple dish smells when you're preparing it for a low-fat, low-calorie Saturday lunch. The aroma is guaranteed to fetch any man in a one-acre radius.

"I slice three or four green bell peppers and rinse the seeds away. One medium-sized yellow onion will do, or two, if you think the balance is better. I smash one or two garlic cloves under the blade of a wide knife so the paper comes off easily.

"I place all the ingredients into a deep saucepan together with virgin olive oil. Onions first, peppers and garlic layered on top, over a low flame, lid on. If there's a tomato in the house, I slice it up and add it at the end, turning off the heat and replacing the lid. Salt and pepper are added at the table. I serve it with crusty Italian bread. It's ultra-delicious, nutritious, and inexpensive."

(TDC: These days, I take a pass on the Italian bread.

Maybe I'll have a WASA bread.)

Again, there's a delicious, inexpensive, low calorie, nutritious lunch. And not a sign of meat. Think about it for a minute, and compare it to what many of us eat for lunch, especially those poor souls away from home, who end up in some fast-food chain restaurant scarfing down a greasy cheeseburger, French fries and an ersatz milkshake filled with trans-fatty acids and sweeteners.

Twenty-first Century Chicken Broth

I think every family has a recipe for chicken soup that's better than anyone else's. Most of them were developed for people living in a different age, so in consideration of our new lives it might be wise to re-visit the original recipes and see what smart homemakers are doing to bring them up to date. Here is my wife's latest recipe—latest not because she is discovering new ways to make it richer and more delicious, but because it is evolving toward a sparer, healthier recipe. It's not her mother's, and it may not be as rich as your mother's chicken broth, but like a lot of things in this book, it's a case of "less is more"—less fat and more health. You might call it space-age chicken broth.

White meat (chicken breast) is less fatty, but whatever parts of the chicken you decide to use, skin it and pull off or slice away all the visible fat before cooking. Put it in a large, deep saucepan with an onion, some chunks of carrot, some celery including the leaves, a couple of garlic cloves, and water to suit. If you include the bones of the chicken, add a teaspoon of vinegar to help dissolve the calcium out of the bones and into the broth.

Start it going over a slow flame, with the lid tilted. When it starts to bubble a bit, reduce the flame even more and simmer it until the chicken is cooked and tender. Add parsley, salt and pepper to taste.

The twenty-first century part of this preparation is not the ingredients, or the cooking time, or its family heritage, but is in removing all of the fat after it's cooked. It's not enough to skim visible fat with a spoon or ladle. The best way to remove most of the fat is to prepare the broth in advance and then either refrigerate it overnight or place it in the freezer (sans meat) long enough to solidify the fat but not long enough to freeze the broth solid. Over the space of an hour or two, virtually all of the fat will come to the surface and congeal. It is nearly all saturated fat—saturated fat is solid at room temperature, remember? If you time it right, the freezer will make the fat firm enough to actually remove in a large sheet leaving only the soup.

Does removing every last bit of the fat remove some of the flavor? Sure it does, but we're about nourishment and health here, not comforting ourselves with ultra-delicious chicken soup like Mama used to serve to the men when they came in from the north forty, where they had been pulling up tree stumps all day.

If you cannot prepare the broth in advance, another way to remove almost all of the fat is with a fat separator, a small pitcher designed for the purpose with a specially-shaped spout that allows the broth to be decanted without including the floating fat. They're sold in every kitchen shop, and are inexpensive. After the broth is poured off, the fat that remains in the separator is discarded before the container is re-filled for the next go. It doesn't remove as much of the fat as freezing the broth, but it works well enough if you're careful.

Serve the chicken broth with the vegetables that were cooked in it, or with raw spinach leaves dropped into it, or blanched escarole. Adding a little raw tomato at the end, so it's just heated by the broth, makes it colorful and more nourishing. If you are serving it as broth, add fresh Italian parsley for garnish and flavor.

One vegetable I've never seen outside Italian kitchens is escarole. Why, I don't know. It is a really delicious, sturdy variety, either blanched using the method outlined above and placed in broth, or eaten raw in a salad. It is wonderful

cooked with white beans, garlic and olive oil and a trace of
hot red pepper. (If you don't think you should eat the beans,
push them aside like my S.O. does. Their flavor will remain
in the greens whether you eat them or not.) It is delicious as
a quick evening meal, served with chicken broth and small
white-meat turkey meatballs. As a salad green, the central
leaves are the best of the best; crunchy, solid, and watery-
moist. Rinsed and placed in a bowl raw with some radicchio,
and a little thin-sliced red onion, sliced cucumber, olive oil,
apple cider vinegar, garlic, salt and pepper and oregano, it is
almost a meal in itself.

Little Low-Fat Meatballs

For that light dinner mentioned above, my S.O. makes
tiny meat balls of ground turkey breast. The breast meat is
lower in fat than ordinary ground turkey, as is turkey meat
itself when compared to chicken. She serves them in the
chicken broth with blanched greens.

Here's the recipe.

Using wet hands, (believe it or not it makes
the cooked meat balls more tender and moist)
she rolls ground white meat turkey into
meatballs a little smaller than an inch in
diameter, and then she browns them lightly in a
non-stick pan with a few drops of olive oil and a
pinch of salt and pepper. Nothing is added to
the meat except perhaps chopped Italian parsley.
With careful handling they stay together, and
she drops them into the broth before serving it.

Portobello Mushrooms and Peas

Slice three or four Portobello mushroom caps
into half-inch wide strips.

Cut up some red onion (or in fact, any onion)
and place it in a large skillet over low to medium
heat with a little olive oil. Add a pinch of salt and

pepper if desired.

When the onion is transparent, add the mushroom caps. If washed before cooking, they produce a watery broth, so unless you like it that way, leave the lid off, or wipe the soil off the mushrooms without using water, like the TV cooks do. Add some garlic and parsley.

When the mushrooms are nearly cooked, add a box of frozen baby peas and continue the cooking over a low heat until the peas are just beginning to get tender.

Serve with a mixed salad. The dish is hearty enough to serve as a main course. It's low in calories and carbohydrates, and is extremely low in fat. Fresh peas have a glycemic index of about 42. If you take two hydroxy-citric acid caps a half-hour before dinner you shouldn't have a problem. Skip the bread.

Fish in the Oven

Use boneless salmon, flounder, codfish, scrod, or other fillet. The recipe is simplicity itself. Dribble a little olive oil in a baking pan lined with aluminum foil, arrange the fillets in the pan, and spread sliced tomatoes on them, along with parsley, fine-chopped garlic (optional, but it shouldn't be), a little more olive oil, salt, pepper, and a little paprika or Old Bay seasoning if desired. Bake at 350 degrees until the fish is flaky, about 10 to 12 minutes. For variety, the tomatoes can be replaced with lemon slices. Near the end, you can sprinkle on some chopped or slivered almonds and toast them by switching to the broiler for one minute. If your oven's like mine, with heating elements top and bottom you don't even need to move the fish. The recipe is low fat, very low in calories, essentially free of carbohydrates, and contains a healthful portion of cholesterol-lowering fish oils.

Ratatouille

Here's my version of the great French and Italian vegetable dish. Cut up a medium to large onion into small chunks, smash five or six cloves of garlic and dice them, slice up two large bell peppers, one or two small Italian egg plants, and three zucchini. Open a large can of whole imported San Marzano plum tomatoes. Place the onion and garlic in a large pan with olive oil and melt the onions a bit. Then add the peppers and simmer until the peppers just start to become tender. Add the sliced zucchini and the egg plant, a little more oil as desired (or none for that matter), some salt, pepper, and fresh basil. Add about half of the can of tomatoes with some of the liquid. Cover and cook a few more minutes. If it looks a little watery, leave the cover off at the last.

It's hearty enough as a main dish for dinner. It keeps well in the fridge, and is delicious cold. If you have a kitchen "boat motor" (hand-held blender), you can puree it into a delicious cold drink.

You can use fresh tomatoes instead of canned, but be careful to add water lest the ratatouille dries out during cooking.

A Really Hearty Dish

Here's a wonderfully tasty soupy stew that my S.O. prepares for a one-dish meal. It's made with "Italian" chicken or turkey sausage, homemade chicken broth, cannellini beans and escarole, with a little added tomato and garlic.

Turkey or chicken sausage comes on packages of six links, and is available in most markets in several varieties. Choose the Italian style sausages for this recipe. Cut up the links into 1-inch pieces, and over a low flame, brown them in a little olive oil in the bottom of a cast-iron cook pot, or other large pot with a thick bottom, until they are nicely browned. Add 14 ounces of chicken broth (You can either buy it, or make it using the recipe described above. Guess which has less chemicals and salt, and no MSG?). To this, add 2 garlic cloves, and 2 large , 14 oz. cans of drained and rinsed cannellini beans. Add three or four tomatoes out of a large can of imported tomatoes, and break them up. After it all begins to simmer again, add a lot of well-rinsed and cut-up escarole and put a lid on the pot for two minutes of simmering. That's it.

Notice that there is no added salt. The turkey sausages have plenty, and if you opt for buying the chicken broth, the dish will actually be too salty, so choose the sodium-free variety if it's available. This is a really delicious soup, and is so hearty that it is adequate as a main course. Let the rest of the family have most of the beans, you take more greens instead and only a few cannellini. It will be just as delicious.

Chapter summary; things to think about

Fabiola's peppers and Onions
Space-Age Chicken Broth
Escarole
Little low-fat meatballs
Portobello mushrooms and peas
Fish in the oven
Ratatouille
Fabiola's turkey-bean soup

23

More Food Preparation Tips, Missing Carbs

Counting missing carbohydrates

If you have decided to count your carbohydrate intake instead of calories, I want to bring up a helpful trick. I call it "counting missing carbohydrates". Every time you consider eating a particular food item and decide against it, look up the carbohydrates you didn't consume. It provides a supportive boost to your morale, and reinforces your determination to continue on.

It's nice to be able to refuse a slice of bread and say to yourself, "There go twenty grams of carbohydrate I didn't eat!" In fact it becomes self-perpetuating. You will find yourself comparing the carbohydrates you ate with those you passed up, and you'll be feeling good about it. It's really important not to tell people that you're doing it, for vocalizing it reduces its power, and can end up serving as a substitute for actually doing it. Just go with feeling good. Soon enough, friends and family will start to look twice, and wonder how you got so svelte when nobody was looking.

In talking about the Krebs cycle, and how exercise activates it, I think I mentioned that before it kicks in, we have to burn off the immediately-available sugar in the bloodstream. Well if you don't eat that slice of bread, it's that much less blood glucose that you have to burn off before getting at some body fat.

If you are interested in what you are putting into your system, and are counting carbohydrates, you will soon learn the carbohydrate content of common foods, like a slice of bread, an apple, a (God forbid!) donut, and the like, so you won't have to continue to look them up.

You don't have to be precise. British school children have a saying, "Best is the enemy of good". If a slice of bread is 22 carbohydrates, round it off to twenty. It's close enough. If you feel like you must, round something else upwards a little to balance it out, but why bother? You need to simplify, and make the counting and memorizing easy, so they provide encouragement, not an arithmetic test.

For a snack, eat vegetables, or free foods, instead of starchy foods. Take a pass on those little bags of processed fruits, nuts and pellets that are sold in gas stations and convenience stores, and are supposed to be "healthy" for us because they have a green name like "Trail Mix", or "Energy Bar", as though we were all trudging ten miles along a mountain trail and needed some kind of special nourishment.

Get yourself in the habit of thinking first of free foods. Try two or three radishes, a small plum tomato, a stalk or two of celery, a small carrot, or a wedge of fennel or celery heart, and then drink a big glass of water. Yes, you can carry them with you in a plastic bag, so no excuses!

I remind those who say that carrots and tomatoes are sugary to remember what they are replacing with these nourishing fiber-foods. But to be on the safe side, just be careful about the amounts.

Cooking greens

Spinach, escarole, Swiss chard, and other cooked greens are a must in any sensible weight-losing diet. Unless they are added to soups, where they are just dropped in at the appropriate time, they should be cooked without a lot of added water. With a tight lid on the saucepan, the water that clings to the greens after washing them is often adequate. If not, add only two or three ounces (an inch or two in the bottom of a kitchen tumbler). Before you place the greens in the pot, very briefly sizzle one or two cloves of crushed or chopped garlic in a little extra-virgin olive oil in the pot. Keep the flame extra-low for this part, so the garlic doesn't brown or burn.

It is suggested that collard greens, kale, rob-broccoli, and the other more-hearty greens be completely covered with water and slowly cooked for about forty-five minutes. My S.O. is not so sure. She cooks them only a little longer than the lighter-weight greens—just until they are tender, and in only about an inch of water. You can serve them the same as the leafier greens, with garlic and oil, and added lemon juice. For a delicious and hearty one-dish meal, you can add into the cooked pot of greens a drained and rinsed can of cannellini beans, red kidney beans, black beans, or chick peas. I like mine with a little ground red pepper. Well-cooked, crumbled bacon makes them even better. Again, when dishing out your own portion, take more greens than beans! And take two hydroxycitric acid caps before you eat.

Sweet potatoes and yams contain a little less available sugar than white potatoes, and a lower glycemic index. And they are rich in fiber, potassium, and beta carotene.

Acorn squashes are full of beta-carotene, and are low in calories. Cut them in two down the middle and bake them in a 350° oven until tender. Cinnamon or nutmeg makes them irresistible. Be careful!

When cooking broccoli, cauliflower, zucchini, green beans, etc. on the stove-top with the lid on, you do not have to cover the vegetables with water. Add just enough to keep them from scorching.

Egg plant has a very low glycemic index, and is a versatile vegetable for any number of baked dishes, some of which are garnished with tomato sauce (the homemade kind described in this chapter). Mint leaves compliment eggplant.

An Eggplant Salad

Boil eggplant quarters in water to which a little vinegar has been added. Boil only until tender. Remove from the pot and skin them by sliding a knife between skin and pulp. Cut them into bite-size pieces and place the pieces into a bowl with lemon juice and olive oil and top with mint leaves. Serve the dish cold.

Italian tomato sauce

I want to say a few words about Italian tomato sauce. Most Americans think that there are two options for what we have come to refer to as "spaghetti sauce". Either the "traditional" kind, consisting of tomatoes, basil and olive oil, and often sugar or wine, simmered for two or three hours in a huge pot full of meatballs, chicken or sausage—or the "other" kind, that we buy at the market in jars. Many choose the latter because it's quick. Heat it up, and depending on the severity of your glucose intolerance, dump it over cooked pasta, and presto! A dish of good stuff.

But wait a minute. Perhaps we should read the table of ingredients before we buy that jar, or better still read the ingredient list on all the popular brands of pasta sauce arrayed along the grocer's shelf. I think you will discover that along with chemical preservatives to increase shelf-life, many brands contain sugar, and/or cornstarch, or often both. And some have monosodium glutamate (MSG), which you will find disguised as "hydrolyzed protein" in the ingredients list.

Is our only other option Mama's traditional, long cooked "spaghetti sauce"?

Not necessarily.

There is another choice, the *real* Italian version—light, healthy, quick to prepare, more nourishing, all natural, much tastier in my opinion, and more versatile. It is a sauce so simple to prepare, and so tasty, that I can't understand why it has escaped the attention of so many American households.
It is fresh tomato sauce as the Italians in Italy prepare it. It doesn't contain cornstarch or preservatives, it's not gooey or pasty. It isn't cooked for two hours. And it contains no added sugar.

> *Note: this is not to say that there is anything wrong with homemade, long-cooked tomato gravy with meats of various kinds. In moderate quantities, it has its place in a normal diet. It is just not for us diabetics, or for people who are trying to lose weight. It contains too much of the wrong kind of fat. And if you add them (we don't), the sugar and red wine don't help either.*

The Recipe

I know you've probably heard this before, but the versions that I see on television always seem to have green peppers in them, or meat of some kind, and those ingredients, tasty though they may be, simply are not marinara sauce. So here is the recipe for Italian marinara sauce.

Vine-ripe tomatoes, either plum-shaped or regular, are cut up into a saucepan seeds and all (for the fiber), unless you hate them and like to fuss. And with the tomatoes, quantity to suit your taste—extra-virgin olive oil, fresh garlic, fresh or dried basil and a little salt. Lightly stir the ingredients together in the saucepan and heat over a low to medium flame just until the tomatoes are cooked—no longer. Because it cooks so quickly, it is a dish that has to be watched. Don't accept phone calls unless you turn off the flame. When the tomatoes have been cooked a few minutes, and begin to soften, you can crush them right in the pot with a potato masher, or just mash them with a fork against the side of the pot. Add the basil at the end.

What do we do in the winter when fresh tomatoes are unavailable or simply awful? My S.O. buys imported San Marzano Italian tomatoes in a can. The best brands do not contain tomato juice or tomato puree, just plain whole plum-shaped tomatoes in their own juices with a little basil. She looks for the Cento™ brand because the label specifies that the contents are San Marzano tomatoes packed in San Marzano, Italy. Cento sells other types of canned tomatoes so read the label carefully.

Its Uses

Among other uses, homemade tomato sauce is delicious over cooked pasta, rice, tofu, eggplant, zucchini, asparagus, green peppers, and baked chicken and fish. You can even saute' it with scrambled eggs for a delicious low-carb treat. For our purposes we will skip the pasta, but you can bake some white-meat turkey meatballs in the oven and place them into the tomato sauce for your meat course. We'll leave the pasta for our children to enjoy when we're away from the house, or out on our walk. Firm, or extra-firm tofu, cut into small cubes, is a good low-calorie substitute for pasta (see below). A plateful has only three grams of carbohydrate. Add a can of drained, packed-in-water tuna to the tomato sauce at the very end of cooking, for variety.

If eggplant is sliced thinly, spread out on a large cookie sheet and placed into a 300 degree oven to soften for a few minutes, then cooled and layered into a baking dish with homemade tomato sauce and basil leaves and some grated imported pecorino cheese (Locatelli Romano is a good brand), or imported parmigiano, (but leave out the mozzarella, because its quantity in baked dishes is such that it represents quite a dose of saturated fat, and it is higher in carbohydrates than other cheeses), you will have a quick, low-calorie, low fat eggplant parmigiano. Please don't buy either of these cheeses if they are not imported from Italy. Domestic "parmesan" cheese is awful—even the name is embarrassing. And domestic pecorino? Don't even ask.

Tofu

If you haven't yet discovered extra-firm tofu, you are in for a surprise. It's good, and good for you. It's so low in carbohydrates that it's almost a free food. It can substitute for pasta, it can be sautéed in a pan, or dashed with cornmeal and toasted in the oven. A brief look for tofu recipes in your web-browser's search engine will reveal literally hundreds of recipes.

In my experience, the simplest ones are the best for diabetics and weight watchers. Some recipes contain honey, maple syrup and other sweeteners. Not necessary. My S.O. buys firm or extra-firm tofu. She prepares the Italian tomato sauce described above, slices the tofu into dice-sized cubes with a sharp wet knife, heats them in a pan, and serves them in the sauce with a little pecorino or parmigiano cheese. A plate full of the little cubes contains about three grams of carbohydrates, and is almost as enjoyable as short pasta, like penne or ziti. The same amount of real pasta provides forty two grams of carbs. Some difference! It provides a great way to enjoy "pasta" without paying the price of added calories and a big spike in your blood sugar.

If the tofu seems to produce too much water when it's cooked, wrap it in a towel before you cut it up and place a can of food or a plastic bag of dried beans on it to press out the water. This is not really necessary though, heating the cubed tofu in an uncovered pan evaporates most of the water.

How to prepare fresh basil leaves for storage

Instead of crushed basil in a shaker jar you can buy fresh basil, or grow it in a flower pot on a sunny porch, and store the leaves in the freezer until needed. Simply strip the leaves off the stems, rinse them a bit and lay them out on a towel to dry off. Then place them loosely in a container with a tight lid, and freeze them. When they're dropped into a pot or dish, they defrost at once and the flavor and aroma are released.

You may have noticed that I include some starchy foods like tomatoes, yams, sweet potato, beans, shredded wheat, and oatmeal in this chapter. It is not a lapse of memory or a "flip-flop". I know only too well what we are dealing with, but if you are exercising regularly, the sugar they contain is not nearly as important a danger as inactivity is, and too much self-denial can lead to rebound eating. We can always "gird our loins", with a couple of hydroxycitric acid caps a half-hour before eating. Too, the balanced nutrition these foods provide is important.

And along those lines, eat a third of a banana once in a while. Leave the rest in its skin in the bowl with the other bananas. It won't go bad, and you can eat another third the next day, and finish it off on the third day. Or place it in the fridge. Can you resist gobbling down the entire banana at one go? I'll leave that to you.

Here's the final food tip of this chapter. NEVER, EVER go into rest stops on a turnpike or parkway for anything but gasoline or to take a "rest"! Eating *anything* in those places is suicide.

Chapter summary; things to think about

Counting Missing Calories
Cooking greens
A Free-Food reminder
Real Italian tomato sauce
Some foods to prepare with it
How to keep fresh basil fresh

24

Vitamin supplements

There is a great deal of information available today on the subject of vitamin supplements. I don't know exactly why, but the very mention of vitamin supplements in amounts exceeding the so-called "recommended daily allowance", or RDA, triggers head-shaking and finger-wagging. Professional people hold strong views on the subject, some dismissing the idea of taking supplements as an utter waste of money, others holding that unsupervised vitamin consumption is not only unsound, but is actually dangerous. I even heard one noted medical authority say that Americans have the most expensive urine in the world, implying that vitamins in excess of the minimum daily requirements are processed straight out of our systems by the kidneys, and are therefore a waste of money.

But not everybody feels this way. As time passes we're beginning to see more light directed at the ever-growing field of nutritional medicine. We are learning that the traditionalists are not without chinks in their armor. Here's a classic example.

The Ascorbic Acid Story

In 1747, James Lind, a Scottish naval surgeon, observed that eating limes or lemons cured shipboard scurvy. Lind published his findings as "Treatise on the Scurvy" in 1753, and by 1795 (almost a half-century later!) all British seamen were given a daily ration of the juice of lemons or limes, ending the long history of shipboard scurvy.

In 1912, a Polish chemist, Vladimir Funk, discovered what he thought was the anti-scorbutic substance in lemons and limes, but it wasn't until 1932, two decades later, that ascorbic acid itself was discovered. Nutritionists and home-economists dominated the research effort at the time, and ran test after test to find the smallest amount of vitamin C that would prevent scurvy, the so-called "minimum daily requirement". The data from their research suggested that 60 milligrams of vitamin C per day would achieve the goal.

Until very recently, there has never been a single long-term test to determine the level of ascorbic acid necessary not just to prevent scurvy, but for optimal health. And the data from that 1932 research are still the basis for the "recommended daily allowance" (RDA) of vitamin C. That's why you may read on a bottle of vitamins that the RDA of vitamin C is 60 mg. A few generous souls have recently allowed as how it is safe to take 90 or even 120 milligrams a day.

I'm sorry, but despite the opinions of people in a position to know better, but who instead, grasp at any shred of "evidence" to show that larger amounts of vitamins are harmful, in today's stressful world I consider that 1932 research outdated and irrelevant.

Because their diet does not provide enough ascorbate (vitamin C) for their needs, many carnivores like dogs, wolves, and predatory cats, produce their own. It turns out that the 60 milligrams recommended for humans is at least 300 times less than the amount of vitamin C produced endogenously each day by meat-eating mammals for their own needs. Carnivores produce 2000 to 3000 milligrams (two to three grams) of vitamin C every day of their lives because there is too little in their regular diet.

Is it possible that buried away in this little fact there might be a message for human beings? We're mammals too. As omnivores on a red meat binge of epic and history-making proportions, do we, in our regular diets, ingest two to three grams of vitamin C every day? You know better.

Traditionalists say that just because other mammals manufacture two or three thousand milligrams of ascorbic acid to meet their daily needs, there is no proof that humans need as much. True enough, but since no one has forwarded *any* research showing that we *don't* need more than sixty milligrams for optimum health, and the fact that there is evidence to the contrary in the studies of Linus Pauling and others, in my view, that argument has no validity at all. And based on their now-proven capacity to retard macular degeneration and cataracts in humans, I am going to continue to take and recommend mega-amounts of vitamin C and the other anti-oxidants found in certain supplements.

Macular degeneration: damage or death of cells in the central part of the retina called the macula lutea—it is the part of the retina that has the most acute visual perception. It is what we use when we look at things directly. All the remainder of the retina is for peripheral vision. There is a higher incidence of macular degeneration in diabetics, in the aged, in hypertensives, and in the presence of some other diseases.

The diagnosis of cataract is made when the lens of the eye loses its clarity. It is not a "film" over the eye, as we often hear. The crystal-clear substance of the eye's lens becomes progressively less clear, and as a result, vision becomes blurred; cataracts are common in the aging eye and in

> *diabetics, among others.*

Along with a few other doctors in my acquaintance, for some twenty five years now, I have been advising my adult patients, especially diabetics, to take a combination of anti-oxidant vitamins to help prevent macular degeneration, to retard formation of cataracts, to slow general aging processes at the cellular level, and to preserve the integrity of cartilage and collagen.

Those of us who have championed mega-amounts of vitamins are finally seeing our views validated by a recent surge of research into cellular aging, collateral damage at the cellular level caused by metabolic oxidation, and the role that anti-oxidants play in retarding that damage. It is now commonly believed that mega-doses of anti-oxidants help prevent cancer and some other diseases, by aiding in the breakdown and elimination of cellular toxins and free radicals.

Perhaps in the Garden of Eden, or some other ideal world, we humans could obtain all the nutrients we require from the food that we eat. Unfortunately such a diet is simply not available in the modern world. In addition to the food we prepare ourselves in our own kitchens, a large part of the American diet is commercially prepared comfort-food, junk food snacks, and adulterated food products for home preparation.

Anti-oxidant Vitamins and where to buy them

Here below is a list of anti-oxidants I recommend and where to buy them.

Vitamin C: 1,500 mg to 3,000 mg a day. That's one and   a half to three grams.
Beta Carotene: 30 to 40,000 int'l units (IU) a day. Beta - carotene is water-soluble, and is not known to alter liver function tests, as oil-soluble carotenes do.
Vitamin E: 400 IU a day

Zinc: 25 mg a day
Selenium: 100 micrograms (mcg) a day
Riboflavin: 50 mg a day
Chromium: 200 mcg a day (double it for diabetics)
Lutein: 20,000 mcg a day
Rutin: 100 mcg a day
Lycopene: 40 mg a day

Note: mcg = microgram, mg = milligram

Fortunately, if you decide to take these vitamins, you do not have to swallow a handful of pills and capsules every day. There are several formulations on the market that provide the entire array in a single capsule. The one I take is *Twinlab® Ocuguard Plus.* In addition to providing the vitamins in the list, four capsules a day (two with breakfast and two with dinner), also supply a citrus bioflavenoid complex, a small amount of taurine and bilberry extract, each an antioxidant with its own benefits. This, and other similar formulations are available in your local vitamin store or on the web. I take lycopene separately as two 20 mg capsules a day. My family and I also take 2,000 mg of calcium citrate in two divided doses.

Unfortunately, today's world demands that I provide a disclaimer, so here it is. Do not take this or any other vitamin preparation without the advice and approval of your doctor. And read the label. I buy my vitamins at health food stores. For freshness I choose the biggest-selling brands: Twinlab, Solgar, and Vitamin Shoppe brands.

Chapter summary; things to think about

Brief history of the discovery of vitamin C
Recommended daily vitamin allowance vs.
megavitamins
Why megavitamins?
Macular degeneration and cataract
Anti-oxidant vitamins
Some brand choices and sources

25

All About Fats

Fats are important for many biological processes. The integrity of cell membranes, including those of the brain, depends on cholesterol. Fats are involved in the production of antibodies, they act as solvents for the fat-soluble vitamins, A, D, E, and vitamin K, and they aid digestion. But this does not provide a rationale for eating butter, pork fat, and marbled beefsteak. We can get pretty much all the fat our bodies need from unsaturated fats.

Knowing which dietary fats raise LDL cholesterol is a long first step toward controlling its blood level. Dietary saturated fat, trans-fatty acids, and dietary cholesterol, all raise blood cholesterol. Monounsaturated fats and polyunsaturated fats generally do not, and there is evidence that they help to lower total cholesterol, and they most certainly improve HDL levels and the all-important HDL/LDL ratio. We know of no absolute biological need for saturated fats in the human diet.

If you want to understand what to eat, you must understand what not to eat. Here is the information on which fat is which, and which is where. I have bad news and I have good news. I'll give you the bad news first.

Saturated Fats

Saturated fat is found mostly in foods from animals, but some plant products are also rich in saturated fats. Fats from animals—beef, beef fat, veal, lamb, pork, lard, poultry fat, butter, cream, milk, cheeses and other dairy products made from whole milk, all contain saturated fat. As stated elsewhere in this book, nearly all saturated fats are solid at room temperature. These foods also contain cholesterol.

Fats from plants

Coconut oil, palm oil and palm kernel oil (often just called tropical oils), and cocoa butter, all contain saturated fat, but in these sources, the saturated fat is liquid or nearly so at room temperature—none-the-less dangerous because of it, however. They are found in many commercial food products. Read ingredients labels and try to avoid them. They are lethal.

Hydrogenated Fats

These are fats that have been chemically modified, usually to prolong shelf life, or to modify the consistency of commercially-prepared foods. The hydrogenation can be complete or partial. Partial hydrogenation is used in vegetable oils to prolong their storage life. Examples of partially hydrogenated oils are some salad and cooking oils. If you look hard enough, and read carefully enough, the ingredients label on the bottle tells the tale. This is a good reason to use pure olive oil.

Both completely-hydrogenated and partially-hydrogenated oils are especially dangerous for two reasons. First, because their presence in commercially-prepared foods is often disguised in very fine print, buried among the list of ingredients on the package, and second, because partially hydrogenated vegetable oils are used so universally in commercial (and home) deep-fryers for French fries and other deep-fried foods. Along with the American Heart Association, the U.S. Government suggests that the American diet may contain a certain low level of hydrogenated fats. I do too. The amount of hydrogenated fat that I recommend as safe to include in our diets is none.

Please understand that I'm not suggesting that you take the approach of limiting your consumption of these fats, and allowing yourself a small amount of saturated fat just for the sake of taking the easy way, or to accommodate your family's tastes, (you'll end up eating it yourself). Eating a limited amount of saturated fat is what the kind folks at the American Heart Association are recommending

To be fair, their recommendations are not meant for diabetics, but for healthy people, but that said, given today's inactive lifestyle and indulgent diet, how do you think we diabetics and heart patients *got* this way?

Avoid them all like the poisons that they are— saturated, hydrogenated, partially hydrogenated alike. (and trans-fatty acids too, as we'll soon see). I'm not offering you comfort here. I'm concerned with saving your life. If you are to avoid them, you must read the fine print, say "Thanks anyway!" and dig into that broccoli.

Trans-fatty Acids

Naturally-occurring trans-fatty acids are found in small amounts in animal products such as beef, pork, lamb and in butterfat of butter and milk.

> *Trans-fatty acids are also formed during the process of hydrogenating oils when manufacturing margarine, shortening, and cooking oils, and they appear in the foods made with them.*

These foods are a major source of trans-fatty acids in our diet—and partially hydrogenated vegetable oils provide about three-fourths of the trans-fatty acids in the American diet.

Clinical studies show that dietary trans-fatty acids raise total blood cholesterol levels. Some researchers believe that trans-fats raise cholesterol levels even more than saturated fats do. More shocking is the fact that they also tend to raise LDL cholesterol and lower HDL cholesterol, inverting that important ratio.

Here's the worst of it. Because there are no standardized methods to do it, it's difficult to measure the trans-fatty acid content of foods. It's also difficult to evaluate dietary intake, especially long-term intake. Because of trans-fatty acid's many sources, we can only estimate, basing our appraisal on identifying foods that are rich in trans-fatty acid content. In one large group study, the most common sources of trans-fatty acid included *beef, pork and lamb, muffins, cookies, biscuits, margarine, and sliced 'American' white bread.*

Many commercially processed fast foods contain high levels of trans-fatty acids. There are no governmental labeling regulations for fast foods. Here's the stinger; even though they are loaded with trans-fatty acids, fast foods can even be advertised as "cholesterol-free", and "cooked in vegetable oil". What do you think? Do fast food companies take advantage of this loophole? If you *don't* think so, there's a bridge in Brooklyn I'd like to sell you.

I told you most of the bad news about fats. Here's the good news. (You deserve a little, after that.)

Unsaturated fats

Polyunsaturated and monounsaturated fats are the two commonest unsaturated fats. They are found in plants and in their oils, *except for tropical plant oils mentioned above (the fats of which are saturated).* There's not much to say about unsaturated fats that hasn't already been said. We've all heard that they are good for us, and that they even lower cholesterol and help change HDL-LDL ratios. In fact, it almost seems that we should try to eat more of them. I'm here to tell you that you should not.

How to deal with the hype

The truth underlying the hype is that we must have a little fat in our diets, and unsaturated fats are infinitely preferable to saturated fats. That's it. In light of what you've read in this book about actual dietary needs, think it through. It won't be any trouble to add a little unsaturated fat to your diet. Across the spectrum of foods, fats are ubiquitous. You'll have more trouble keeping fats *off* your menu than finding some to eat. Just make sure that whichever you choose is not saturated. If you're in doubt, opt for safety. Skip the fat altogether and choose a different food. It's only for this once, right? What's one little dietary sacrifice in the grand scheme of things?

How's that for a turnabout? A little reverse psychology! Usually, "just this once" involves indulging a weakness. Instead, we are using the rationalization to the opposite effect—to help us to eat less instead of more—or should I say, 'eat better instead of worse'?

Here is how to put it to use; tell yourself that you'll eat some fat later. For now, just eat something safe to take the edge off your hunger—a couple of radishes maybe, or a stalk of celery, or a pickle. Plan to come back later and eat something really tasty. Then don't come back. Interest yourself in something more important.

Polyunsaturated fats—Found in safflower, sesame, and sunflower seeds, corn and soybeans, many nuts and seeds, and their oils.

Monounsaturated fats—These include canola oil, olive oil, peanut oils, and oil from avocados.

Both polyunsaturated and mono-unsaturated fats help lower total blood cholesterol, but mono-unsaturates have been demonstrated to actually increase the proportion of HDL in blood fats. The richest kitchen source is probably olive oil, which has a better ratio of mono-unsaturates to poly-unsaturates than all other oils. Canola oil and peanut oils are also rich in mono-unsaturates.

Below is a list of general dietary recommendations prepared by the American Heart Association, with notes by me in italics. I'm hesitant to provide this list at all, lest you think that because it originates from an authority as reputable as the American Heart Association, the recommendations must be safe. They may be safe for some, but they are not safe for us. That's why it's important for you to know about them. The suggestions will remind us of where, and who particularly, we are, and why we cannot just apply such suggestions to ourselves without thoughtful analysis. The list was designed for healthy individuals, so they can avoid or postpone the types of health problems described in this book, the health problems that prompted me to write it and you to read it, because we likely already have some of them. Please bear this in mind as you read down the list.

One more thing. I'm not commenting on the items just to be a wise guy, or to make an attempt at being funny, but to drive home a few important points, and to encourage you to analyze everything you read from the standpoint of whether what *you* choose to eat is safe, and nourishing for *you,* and not because some "authority" tells you it's okay.

Here, in their own words, is the American Heart Association list: (My comments are italicized.)

1. Use naturally occurring, un-hydrogenated oil such as canola or olive oil when possible. *(Not 'when possible' - always!)*

2. Look for processed foods made with un-hydrogenated oil rather than hydrogenated or saturated fat. *(Do not eat processed foods, period! They are what got us here.)*

3. Use margarine as a substitute for butter, and choose soft margarines (liquid or tub varieties) over harder stick forms. Shop for margarine with no more

than 2 grams of saturated fat per tablespoon and with liquid vegetable oil as the first ingredient. Look for those labeled "trans-fat free." *(Aside from providing a tasty, salty grease, there is no reason for butter or margarine of any type in your diet. However, I think that after you have gotten down to fighting trim, one of the new "cholesterol-lowering" tub margarines is safe enough in small amounts. The trouble is that when you decide to add margarine to your diet, you have to put it on something don't you? There's the rub.)*

4. French fries, doughnuts, cookies and crackers are examples of foods that are high in trans-fatty acids. Consume them infrequently. *(Consume them never! They are killers!)*

5. Limit the saturated fat in your diet. If you don't eat a lot of saturated fat, you won't be consuming a lot of trans-fatty acid. *(I would only preface the first word "Limit", with "Severely".)*

6. Eat commercially fried foods and commercial baked goods infrequently. Not only are these foods very high in fat, but that fat is also likely to be very hydrogenated, meaning a lot of trans-fatty acids. *(Again – do not eat ANY commercially-prepared fried foods or fast foods of any kind, including "buttered" movie-theatre popcorn, which just might be the worst offender.)*

7. Commercial shortening and deep-frying fats will continue to be made by hydrogenation and will contain trans-fatty acids. That's just one more reason to eat fried fast-food infrequently. *(Infrequently? Why eat it at all?)*

8. The American Heart Association recommends that people limit trans fats to less than 2 grams per day. *(What? Given the increasingly gloomy outlook on diabetes and heart disease numbers in our country, this is an irresponsible recommendation.)*

More than you bargained for:

Federal regulations allow food labels to say that there are zero grams of trans fat in a grocery-shelf food product *as long as there's less than half a gram of trans fats per serving.* (Note that it is "per serving", not "per package".) And most, if not all packages contain more than one serving. So what happens? We open the package and eat two or three of the goodies inside. Result? Another load of artery-clogging trans fats.

The way to find out if "zero trans fats" *means* none at all, or the half-gram per serving allowance, is to read the ingredients list. If you see "partially hydrogenated fat" anywhere in the list, assume that the product contains trans-fats. Partially hydrogenated oils are the primary source of trans-fats.

The reason that the half-gram threshold was adopted is because it is difficult to measure low levels of fat content in food products. You should be aware that the same half-gram allowance is made for saturated fats as well. When we eat that microwave popcorn that boasts "zero trans fats per serving", there are also "zero grams" of saturated fats. Eat more than "one serving"? You're on your own in a dangerous world. And I've said nothing here about restaurant and coffee-shop foods, like muffins, Danish, cake, commercial pies, etc. Just so you know, *one store-bought or coffee shop muffin contains more saturated fat than two eggs.*

Chapter summary; things to think about

The importance of dietary fats, their biological functions.
Types of fats, their food sources and properties explained
of trans-fatty acids; the hidden trans-fats in junk food and commercially-prepared foods
American Heart Association's general dietary recommendations with added comments for diabetics and people trying to lose weight
A warning about hidden trans fats and saturated fat content of prepared foods

26

Programs and Approaches

Nearly all books on diabetes, and related conditions like obesity, discuss to greater or lesser degree, a multitude of treatment modalities. That is to say, dietary, medicinal, and weight-control measures necessary for the control of the several degrees of severity of Type II diabetes. For example, glucose intolerance controlled by reducing sugar intake alone, diabetes controlled by significant weight loss, diabetes controlled by diet and medication, and so on.

Without discussing diabetic medicines, I would like to outline a two-pronged approach to improving your diabetes that will benefit individuals in all of the above categories. Despite it's great benefits, it is simplicity itself. After a few weeks, you will wonder what all the fuss is about on TV, with weight machines, platforms, rocking chairs, big rubber balls, trampolines, "six-pack" ab devices, and so on. (In case you haven't figured it out yet, it's all about money.)

In the beginning, continual close medical consultation will be necessary, because changing your diet and increasing your activity level will alter your body chemistry, especially your glucose metabolism. The alterations will be for the better.

First efforts should be directed at controlling your diet,

coupled with an exercise program that starts easy, and advances in difficulty to suit your individual abilities, as they relate to your age, body weight, and the presence of other medical conditions. When daily exercise, and a healthful diet are well in place, the overall control of blood sugar will be much easier, and should be attainable with lower amounts of medication. Sometimes, when the glucose intolerance is not too severe, medications can be eliminated entirely be means of a vigorous exercise campaign coupled with a careful diet.

Even if your particular case is beyond this stage, regular exercise and a proper diet will help level out plasma glucose numbers, making steady control much easier to maintain. This is of paramount importance, because as I've stated, if they are frequent enough, even small elevations in blood sugar can have deleterious systemic effects over time.

An Easy Exercise Plan

Set a Fast-Walking Course. Two Methods

1. Using time as a guide, go out tomorrow morning and try to walk a circular route that will start and finish at your abode. Walk as rapidly as you can, but not so fast that you become out of breath or uncomfortable. If a circuit is geographically impossible, (which is unimaginable to me), walk ten or fifteen minutes out and ten or fifteen minutes back. If you feel more secure staying near home, find a short circuit, perhaps around one city block, or the suburban equivalent. If the route seems too short, you can always go around again. If walking for half an hour is too taxing, walk for fifteen minutes, or even ten minutes, and build your time over the days and weeks. (See #2 below)

2. Distance method; use the odometer in a car to measure off a distance that you think you can walk, starting and ending at your home. In the city, it can be four or five city blocks, in the country, a half-mile, a mile, or two miles, depending on your physical condition and age. Again, if you

start with a short route you can always make two circuits when you become fitter, or change the route altogether.

Fast-walk the route briskly every Monday, Wednesday, and Friday. Head up, chest out, shoulders back. Take the longest strides you comfortably can, even if you think it looks funny. No one will care or pay any attention at all, beyond thinking, "There goes a walker."

Look in my menu list, and choose a breakfast and a lunch. There isn't much variety, but what's the difference? Your life doesn't have to revolve around food. Remember the goal, and the ultimate role of utilizing food as fuel and not as a source of emotional comfort. The food we eat, of course, is much more than mere fuel, but it helps you cut down on intake to think of it in these terms. If you work, and have to eat out, eat a restaurant salad for lunch or a veggie burger with a salad on the side. No bread, crackers, or roll please. And no ketchup. Out of sight is out of mind, so ask the server not to bring bread to your table. And for the same reason, hand off the saltines to the server before you start to eat. Be careful which salad dressing you select. I have been looking for a long while, and I've yet to find any prepared dressings that are safe for diabetics, and people with a weight problem. Even if they say "diabetic" on the label, that means only that they are lower in sugar than the company's regular dressing, or that they use an artificial sweetener in place of sugar to keep your taste buds habituated. And our commercial food suppliers do not (or will not) understand that sugar is only one of the dietary dangers; most bottled dressings contain hydrogenated fats and trans-fatty acids as well.

Vinegar and oil, garlic, or oregano, and salt and pepper make the safest and most healthful salad dressing. The waiter will bring the bottles if you ask him or her. And frankly, it tastes great. In gastronomically wonderful Italy, where salads are a part of almost every meal save breakfast, this same dressing, or other home-made dressings poured fresh over the greens are all they ever eat. Even restaurant dressings are prepared fresh at the table, the same combination that you can pour for yourself at the restaurant table where you eat. Commercially bottled salad dressing is a dead dog in Italy.

Whatever you choose to eat for dinner, avoid red meat, potatoes, macaroni, pasta, rice, or dessert. Eat a little broiled or roasted chicken or fish, some tofu, a shrimp stir-fry with broccoli ("fry" because you use a little olive oil to cook it in, not because you deep-fry it), a nice fresh salad, or some other cruciferous vegetable in its place. If you absolutely, positively must have bread, eat a WASA bread, but be warned—think of the smoker. You'll never break the bread habit by "cutting down". If you *must* have an after-meal sweet, have a stick of sugarless chewing gum and a cup of tea with fat-free milk. The hot tea intensifies the sweetness of the gum. Important tip: (and you know why!), leave your kitchen or dining room with your tea, and drink it in another room.

If, after some weeks, your fast walk becomes too easy, or your enthusiasm carries you away, get out the exercise bands and do a few sets of upper body exercises on the days you do not walk. After a time, when every other day becomes too easy, try doing your walking route five or six days a week. Lean into it and walk even faster.

Buy a cheap pedometer clicker, and hang it on your belt. They come with a belt clip, cost less than ten dollars on the web or in drug stores, and are surprisingly informative. It's fun to see that you have walked 7,000 steps over a day's time, and humans being human, it invariably engenders a desire to try for 8,000. They come with a little booklet that tells you how many steps add up to a mile.

Gaining Endurance – How to make the most of it

As excellent as walking is, if you are assiduous in keeping to your routine there will come a time when you may decide it is just not enough. You will want to do something more. Perhaps you find yourself jogging for short distances during your walks, or having the urge to jog but resisting because you are not sure that you should. The urge to run is strong in human beings. It has accompanied us down through the ages, hidden away in our genetic memories just waiting there for a chance to re-assert itself. So if your doctor approves, interrupt your walking with short periods of easy jogging—a short-step, shuffling jog is perfectly adequate as a beginning. It is said to have been employed by the early American Indian to travel long distances on foot. In my little park in New York by the East River, I see ladies and gentlemen getting their daily two miles doing exactly that—arms held close with elbows bent and a look of joy in their eyes.

This is also a good time to add weight training. You can do it with dumbbells, with the elastic stretch bands, or even with cans of tomato or pumpkin or some such. Cans of food are perfectly adequate substitutes for dumbbells, and are available in lots of different weights. See the section in Chapter 19 on weight training, and start doing the routine on the days you do not walk.

Warming Up Routine

Start your session by warming up. Walk around on your toes for about one minute, then do a minute more on your heels, then another 30 seconds or so of lifting your legs high (prancing), then kicking your heels up behind (think about kicking yourself in the butt with your heels), then swinging your arms really high as you walk, then punching the air in front of you as you walk. Then do another 30 seconds of arm curls while walking.

You can do the stretches described below just as soon as you have warmed up your muscles. When you feel that the large muscles in your arms and legs are loose and warm, do the following stretch routine. It starts from a standing position, arms at sides.

Stretching Routine

Stand at ease legs a bit apart and tilt and tilt your head to each side, then forward, then backward, holding each head position for about thirty seconds. In other words bend your neck to your right shoulder, then to your left shoulder, then forward, and backward. At the extreme of each position, push a little. Hold it steadily, then relax a moment before tilting your head in a new direction.

Stretch your arms straight out in front of you loosely interlocking your fingers, then rotate your palms away from you. Hold until you feel shoulders, arms and fingers relaxing.

Holding this stretch, bring your arms straight up above your head. Hold as you did above.

Behind your back, grasp one hand with the other, arms reasonably straight, then push your hands backwards away from your body until you feel a stretch in your shoulders and arms. Hold until you feel the muscles relax.

Stretch your Achilles' tendons using the methods outlined in the chapter on walking. Here it is again, lifted verbatim from that section. Stand two to three foot-lengths away from a tree or lamppost and using it for support, bend your knees a bit and lean forward until you feel a stretch in your Achilles' tendon. Hold it long enough to feel the tendons and calves relaxing. (Doing it one leg at a time allows you to concentrate your mind better).

Groin stretch. To stretch the groin muscles, semi-squat with knees bent and your feet spread almost as wide as you can reach, then lean to the right side, placing your hands down onto your bent right leg, keeping your left leg pretty much straight. If you can, keep the left foot (the "straight-leg" foot) flat on the ground and pointed straight ahead and the bent-leg foot wherever it is comfortable. Then switch sides. Hold each side until you feel your inner thigh and groin muscles stretching out a bit. No leaning on your knee with your hand though it puts unnatural pressures on the joint and patellar cartilage. Support your hands on your thigh. If you need to, hold on to something with one hand; fireplug, sapling, sign post, door frame or counter top if indoors.

Thigh Stretch. Stand beside a chair or some other support and hold one foot up behind you with your hand. Pull it in towards your buttock. Try to keep the knee of the bent leg close beside the leg you're standing on, and feel the pull in your front thigh muscle. Hold until you feel it relaxing, then switch sides.

The above descriptions may sound like stretching is complicated, and that it takes a long time. Describing it here takes longer than doing it. After you understand the moves, you can complete it all in about eight minutes. Stretching is necessary to avoid muscle injury, but don't regard it as a chore. After a few days, when the effects of stretching become apparent to you in better sleep, looser joints and fewer aches and pains, you will look forward to doing it. Some people like it so much that they find ways to develop it into the actual mainstay of their fitness improvement program, perhaps as yoga or tai chi, both of which build core muscle strength, and greatly improve balance, leg strength, and breathing.

Good Luck and Goodbye!

I hope that I have convinced you that these little routines, coupled with a sensible diet, will change your life in absolutely profound ways. I needn't go into the benefits again, but believe me when I tell you that you will really and truly become a different person—inside as well as outside. And the people you love, and who love you, will be grateful.

If you find this book helpful, you may want to order some as gifts for your friends. It could save their lives!

Good luck and God bless! I'm glad we met. Feel free to contact me by email with questions.

My email address: tdeecy@gmail.com

Appendix

APPENDIX A

Digestion of Sugars

Single sugars monosaccharides are digested essentially without digestive action. Monosaccharides are found in honey, some fruits and some vegetables.

Double sugars - disaccharides. Found in table sugar, maple syrup, milk, and some fruits and vegetables. These require some digestive action but not much. Intestinal enzymes quickly break them down.

Complex carbohydrates - polysaccharides. Chains of many single sugars linked together. Found in grains and their products (bread and the like), legumes, rice, pasta, and many vegetables. In the intestine, they require prolonged enzymatic action to be broken down for digestion, hence are favored in diabetic diets because their slower digestion means slower absorption into the blood stream and favors a slow rise in blood sugar with less spiking.

Testing Your Blood Sugar level

A word about when to stick your finger. Whenever I ask an early diabetic what time of day they test their blood glucose they almost invariably tell me that they were instructed to test in the evening, usually before bed. There is only one place they can get this directive, and it's not from their aunt Millie, who also has "a little sugar". It's from their doctor.

If this is the instruction most new diabetics get it is disturbing. Why? Because it is pretty much a waste of time. It provides no information of any value to the patient (or the doctor!) in finding out whether the diabetes is under control. Worse, it very often provides erroneous and unjustified "evidence" that the patient is appropriately controlling their blood sugar.

The only useful home test

Allow me to suggest that the only home test of any value to a person with early to moderate Type II diabetes is a two-hour post-prandial test. Think about it. It's ten-thirty P.M. and you haven't eaten since dinner—probably four to five hours. If you are controlling your glucose intolerance by diet alone or with a prescription medicine, there's a good chance that your sugar will be in the normal range at that hour. If you do a finger-stick two hours after your dinner the result might be an eye-opener because that's when the sugar load of a meal causes the blood sugar to be at its highest. Two-hour post-prandial tests, as they are called, provide the answer to two important questions:

"How is my diet? Am I eating too much sugar and starch for my medicine to control?"

And the obverse,

"Given how much sugar and/or starch I am eating, is my present dose of medicine doing the job?" Sticking your finger at bedtime is usually too long after eating to answer these two questions.

The conclusion is obvious. A two-hour post-prandial blood-glucose test should supplant the bedtime finger stick. And to learn even more about yourself, test it occasionally two hours after breakfast and/or lunch as well.

Counting your Pulse

Place two fingers over your wrist, like they do in the movies, look at the second hand on your watch, and after you locate the steady beating of the radial artery on the thumb side of the palmer surface of your wrist, count the beats for ten seconds. Then multiply by six to get the number of beats per minute. Since there are six units of ten seconds in a minute, the result will be the number of beats in one minute. For a slightly more accurate reading you can count for fifteen seconds and multiply by four, but after you've become skilled at it a ten-second count is precise enough.

Incidentally, you may have been told that you should never take a pulse with your thumb. Why? Because your thumb has a pulse of its own, and you don't want to get an erroneous reading. But this only makes sense when you're taking somebody else's pulse. The pulse in your thumb is synchronous with your other pulses—the carotid pulse in the side of the neck, the radial pulse in your wrist and so on. So when you're taking your own pulse, what's the difference whether you use your thumb or your finger? If it's more comfortable to use your thumb instead of your first two fingers, feel free.

Exercise target pulse rate; simple method

The recommended formula for estimating your target pulse rate is as follows; the *maximum pulse rate* is 220 minus your age, and the *target pulse rate* for a safe pulse rate during or just after completing exercise, is 60 to 80 percent of that.

If you're fifty, subtract 50 from 220, and multiply the result by 80 to get 136. This is a reasonable number to shoot for after you have become fit. If you are seventy, subtract that number from 220 to get 150. Eighty percent of this is 120. Again, a reasonable target for that age.

What Target Pulse Rates Tell Us

Target heart rates are effective in evaluating initial fitness levels and in monitoring higher levels of fitness as you progress through your program. This approach requires measuring your pulse periodically as you exercise, and every few minutes after you stop, to determine how long it takes for your pulse to return to normal. In a previous section, I talked about cardiac stroke volume and how a stronger heart pumps more blood throughout the body with each heartbeat, so that fewer beats per minute are needed. The same mechanism allows the heart to slow down to resting pulse rate sooner after it has been elevated by exercise.

A simple alternative to calculating target heart rates

I mentioned this in the section on walking. It is for people who find that taking their pulse is simply too difficult while they are exercising. The idea behind it is to set a "conversational pace" while walking. If you can talk and walk rapidly at the same time, your heart is not working too hard. If you can sing and maintain your present level of effort, you are probably not working hard enough. If you are not doing either of the above (talking or singing) and get out of breath anyway you are working too hard—especially if you have to stop and catch your breath. The solution of course, is to slow down to the point where you can walk and talk. Although it is not a scientific approach, in the absence of clinical heart disease, this method is a good rough guide. I know that I recommended walking alone instead of taking a stroll with a friend or S.O. If you're afraid you might embarrass yourself by being seen "talking to yourself", talk on your cell phone. And one addendum; if walking alone seems to risky for you because of your health, or even because you find it too lonely, by all means walk with a companion! Walking is supposed to be fun, not punishment.

The table on the next page shows estimated target heart rates for different age categories. If you don't have the patience to check your pulse, or just want to "get in the zone" and enjoy the great outdoors without doing arithmetic, use this chart. Look for the age category closest to yours and read across to find your target heart rate.

The table for reference only, so ask your doctor if the target rate you've picked out for yourself is safe. The age-adjusted maximum heart rates in beats per minute (BPM) are also listed.

Target Heart Rates

Age	Target Rate	Maximum rate
• 20 yrs	100-150	220
• 25 yrs	98-146	195
• 30 yrs	95-142	190
• 35 yrs	93-138	185
• 40 yrs	90-135	180
• 45 yrs	88-131	175
• 50 yrs	85-127	170
• 55 yrs	83-123	165
• 60 yrs	80-120	160
• 65 yrs	78-116	155
• 70 yrs	75-113	150

The figures above are averages, and can be used as general guidelines. Ask your doctor for more specific numbers. A few high blood pressure medications lower the maximum allowable heart rate and change the target zone rate. If you are taking high blood pressure medicine, call your physician and find out if your target rate needs to be different from the age-normal rate.

How to Pace Yourself

When beginning an exercise program, aim at the lowest part of your target pulse rate zone for the first few weeks. Then over time, gradually build up to the higher part of your target zone. After six months or more of regular exercise, depending on your age, you might be able to exercise comfortably up to 85 percent of your maximum heart rate if your doctor approves. But you do not have to exercise that hard to stay fit. Remember the Krebs cycle.

What you can learn from pulse-counting

Ambient heart rate: the measurement when you are sitting and are inactive. It should be around 70 beats per minute (bpm) for most people. In general, the lower your ambient rate, the better. Many world-class athletes have ambient heart rates in the range of 40 to 50 bpm.

Resting heart rate: measured when you first wake up in the morning before you get out of bed. Within reason, the lower the number the better. Resting heart rate numbers range from the 50s to the 70s.

Maximum Heart Rate: the fastest your heart can beat for one minute, age-adjusted. Decreases with age. Maximum heart rate doesn't decrease if you maintain your fitness (it does if you become de-conditioned because you have stopped exercising). To estimate maximum allowable heart rates there are arithmetic formulas. Here is one such formula:

> Age/Weight Predicted Maximum Heart Rate:
> 210 minus 1/2 your age minus 1% of your
> body weight + 4 (males), or + 0 (females)
> An example: say I am a sixty year-old male
> weighing 160 pounds.
> 210 minus 30 (half my age) = 180, minus 1.6
> (1% of my weight) = 178, plus 4 (male) = 182.
> If I were a female I would not add the
> number 4 to the result.

Is it useful to you? Yes, if you want to calculate your target exercise rate on your own. No, if you just need to know it for your exercise program, because the information is widely available elsewhere (e.g. in this Appendix).

Maximal heart rate generally declines with age from about 220 beats per minute in childhood to about 160 beats per minute at age 60. This decrease in the maximum heart rate is fairly linear, falling by approximately 1 beat per minute per year. You or your doctor can do the simple calculation when you have a stress test. Just remember that the age-adjusted maximum heart rate is not the target heart rate that you use when you are exercising.

APPENDIX B:

Reference Information

Glycemic Index of common foods
Breads

White bread	100
Waffle	96
Donut	106
Whole wheat bread	75
Bread stuffing	74
Kaiser roll	73
Bagel, white	72
Melba toast	70
Tortilla, corn	70
Rye bread	75
Whole wheat pita	58
Pumpernickel bread	49

Cereals

Grapenuts	96
Cornmeal (polenta)	98
Shredded Wheat	69
Total (cereal)	86
Puffed Rice	90
Rice Chex	89
Corn Flakes	84
Corn Chex	83
Rice Krispies	82
Grapenut Flakes	80
Cocoa pops	77
Cheerios	74
Puffed Wheat	67
Museli	66
Cream of Wheat	66
Bran Chex	58

Oatmeal	55
Special K	54
All-bran	60
Oat Bran	78

Crackers/Cookies

Vanilla Wafers	77
Rice Cakes	77
Water Crackers	72
Golden Grahams	71
Stoned Wheat Thins	67
Shortbread	64

Dairy

Ice Cream	61
Ice cream, low fat	71
Yogurt, low fat, artificially sweetened	20
Milk, skim	46
Milk, regular 4% fat	39
Yogurt – with sugar	33
Yogurt – sugar free	14

Fruits

Watermelon	100
Apple	54
Banana	77
Cherries	32
Grapefruit	36
Peach, fresh	60
Orange	63
Dried fruit	70
Pineapple	66
Cantaloupe	65
Blueberry	59
Orange juice	57
Mango	55
Fruit cocktail	75
Kiwi	52

Grapes	43
Pear	35
Strawberry	32
Grapefruit	25
Plum	25
Cherries	23

Grains

Rice – instant	88
Millet	71
Rye flour	65
Rice, white	83
Couscous	93
Bran	60
Buckwheat	54
Bulgur	48

Legumes

Lima beans, baby, frozen	46
Chick peas (garbanzo beans)	47
Kidney beans	42
Black beans	43
Navy beans	54
Fava beans	80
Baked beans – canned	68
Black eyed peas	42
Split peas	32
Butter beans	31
Lentils	29
Beans – dried	29
Soybeans	18
Broad beans	113
Pinto beans	55

Pasta

Spaghetti, wheat	53
Elbow Macaroni	64
Brown rice pasta	92

Refined pasta	65
Gnocchi	65
Whole grain pasta, thick	45

Vegetables

Broccoli	10
Cabbage	10
Lettuce	10
Mushrooms	10
Onions	10
Red Peppers	10
Carrots	49
Beets	64
Pumpkin	75
Parsnips	97
Beets	91
Sweet corn	78
Peas, dried	32
Parsnips	97
Potato, baked	121
Potato instant	83
Potato mashed	73
New Potato	62
French fries	75
Sweet potato	77
Yam	51
Pumpkin	75
Rutabaga	72
Carrot	71
Sweet corn	55
Tomato	38
Bean sprouts	low
Cauliflower	low
Eggplant	low
Peppers	low
Squash	low
Plum	55
Peas, green	68

Rice, brown	79

Miscellaneous

Tofu frozen dessert	115
Maltose	105
Glucose	100
Rice cake	82
Jelly beans	80
Pretzels	80
Honey	73
Corn chips	73
Soft drink	70
Angel food	67
Sucrose	65
Hamburger bun	61
Sponge cake	54
Chocolate	49
Fructose	23
Split pea soup	86
Orange juice	74
Apple juice	58
Melba toast	100
Raisins	91
Popcorn 7	9
Waffles	109
Pizza cheese	60
Hummus	6
Peanuts	15
Walnuts	15
Cashews	22

Mgs. of Calcium in usual quantities of foods

1 cup skim milk	302
1 cup 1% low-fat milk	300
1 cup 2% low-fat milk	297
1 cup whole milk	291
1 cup buttermilk	285

1 oz. Swiss cheese	272
1 oz. cheddar cheese	204
1 oz. American cheese	174
1/2 cup 2% cottage cheese	77
1 cup low-fat plain yogurt	415
1 cup low-fat yogurt with fruit	345
3 oz. sardines with bones	345
3 oz. salmon with bones	99
3 oz. shrimp, canned	145
4 oz. tofu, processed with calcium sulfate	145
1 cup oysters	90
1/2 cup cooked collard greens	179
1/2 cup cooked kale	103
1/2 cup bok choy 1	26
1/2 cup cooked turnip greens	126
1/4 of a 14-inch cheese pizza 3	32
1/2 cup macaroni and cheese 1	81
1 cup cream of mushroom soup with milk	191
1 cup cream of tomato soup made with milk	168
1 taco	174
1 cup American cheese	124
1 tbsp. blackstrap molasses	137

Antagonists to Calcium Absorption
- Soft drinks
- High fiber diets
- Coffee
- Excessive amounts of fat
- Sugar
- Salt

About the author:

Thomas D. Cherubini is a retired New York-Presbyterian Hospital/Cornell Medical Center doctor, an ophthalmologist, who, a year before he retired from medical practice, discovered that he had early type II diabetes. In his efforts to fight the disease and return to health, he made some surprising discoveries, which provided the basis for a remarkable improvement of his condition. He knew from his medical practice that most diabetics do not die from their disease. They die instead, from its complications, the most prevalent of which is heart disease, the commonest killer in America.

Out of his research and this knowledge, he developed simple but surprisingly effective dietary and life-style changes that have returned him to health, so he decided to share his knowledge with others via this book. Interestingly, these same methods can help control and reduce body weight, so this book turns out to be just as useful (and important!) for weight-conscious people as for type II diabetics.